Clinical Care Manual for Children's Nursing

edited by
Joanie Barber, Allan Campbell and Liz Morgan

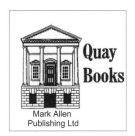
Quay
Books

Mark Allen
Publishing Ltd

Quay Books Division, Mark Allen Publishing Limited, Jesses Farm, Snow Hill, Dinton, Wiltshire, SP3 5HN

British Library Cataloguing-in-Publication Data
A catalogue record is available for this book

© Birmingham Children's Hospital NHS Trust 2000
ISBN 1 85642 128 7

Printed in the UK by The Cromwell Press, Trowbridge, Wiltshire, United Kingdom

Clinical Care Manual for Children's Nursing

Contents

About the editors

Joanie Barber RGN, RSCN is a Staff Nurse working on an orthopaedic and trauma ward. She was formerly a Professional Development and Practice Facilitator.

Allan Campbell RGN, RSCN, BSc (Hons) Health Studies, ENB 100 is a Charge Nurse working in cardiology with an extensive background in intensive care and high dependancy nursing. He has recently undertaken the post of Clinical Placement Co-ordinator/Teacher Practitioner in the education department of the Birmingham Children's Hospital NHS Trust.

Liz Morgan MSc, RGN, RSCN, RCNT, RNT is the Head of Nursing at the Birmingham Children's Hospital NHS Trust.

Acknowledgements

This manual represents a considerable amount of work by a number of nurses and other colleagues, much of which has been undertaken in addition to their normal day-to-day work. Their motivation, commitment and enthusiasm to this project must be acknowledged and admired as the Trust aims to contribute to the delivery of safe and consistent nursing care to children wherever they may be. This manual would not have come about if it were not for their efforts. We would like to thank all members of the existing Clinical Guidelines Group and Sharon Blair for her unfailing patience in typing and amending each guideline numerous times to meet our satisfaction. Thanks must also be extended to members of the previous Procedure Groups at Birmingham Children's Hospital NHS Trust, too numerous to mention and finally to Sue Smallman, currently Professional Officer, Paediatrics, UKCC.

Members of the procedure group

The Clinical Guidelines (Nursing) Group who developed this text:

> Joanie Barber: Staff Nurse, Trauma and Orthopaedics, formerly Professional Development and Practice Facilitator

> Allan Campbell: Charge Nurse, Cardiac Service

> Angela Ledsham: Senior Sister, Intensive Care Unit

> Amanda Whitehouse: Staff Nurse, Cardiac Service

> Elaine Berry : Staff Nurse, General Medicine

> Ruth Bailey: Staff Nurse, Renal Service

> Julie Clissett: formerly Senior Sister, General Medicine

> Sue Philpott: Senior Lecturer in Children's Nursing, University of Central England

> Julie Plant: Senior Nurse Manager, Community Paediatrics

> Jacqui McDaid: formerly Staff Nurse, General Surgery

We would also like to thank the following staff for their help, advice and guidance in developing the format of this text.

> Gail Moore and Carl Beech for production of an audit tool to accompany the Clinical Guidelines.

> Suzan Smallman, formerly Senior Nurse of Professional Development, who was instrumental in setting up the Clinical Guidelines Group.

> Tim Kilner, Senior Lecturer, University of Birmingham, whose knowledge of legal issues and his experience as a nurse practising outside paediatrics brought clarity and encouragement to our endeavours.

In addition, we would like to thank our nursing colleagues who have enabled us to develop this work alongside our clinical role and responsibilities, including Sheila Marriot, Director of Nursing and Liz Morgan, Head of Nursing as well as all the Ward Managers.

Foreword

The Government in *A First Class Service:Quality in the New NHS* (1998) states that clinical decisions should be based on the best possible evidence of effectiveness and all staff should be up-to-date with the latest developments in their field.

The Nursing Clinical Guidelines Group at the Birmingham Children's Hospital NHS Trust has been developing and refining their child health nursing clinical guidelines over the last few years. However, it has been found that there is a limited body of nursing research generated knowledge available on which to base best practice. It is the experience and expertise of clinical nursing staff, plus the available evidence which form the basis of these guidelines. The next piece of work to be done is the development of multi-professional guidelines.

The guidelines are not published as the definitive 'recipe book' for clinical nursing interventions but provide a snapshot in time. Clinical care is constantly changing and the purpose of the book is to provide a foundation of peer-reviewed clinical guidance which is up-to-date at the time of going to press. Ownership of guidelines is likely to be a key component to compliance and guideline evaluation. I would encourage colleagues to use and adapt these guidelines to suit local needs and perhaps involve children and young people in their further development. It is important to obtain feedback from the professionals using guidelines in practice, because acceptance in principle may be mistaken for compliance. Therefore, clinical audit of the guidelines is important and a section has been included to provide a review framework for readers to customise.

In order to assist nurses in the delivery of care, guidelines need to be flexible and take into account the wishes of individual children and young people. Many of the procedures within this book are invasive in nature and psychological preparation and support have been included where appropriate. Although written consent is not required for the implementation of most nursing procedures, nurses have a moral responsibility to respect the rights of the child or young person to give agreement, even when parents or carers provide proxy consent.

In the preparation of nursing guidance, a balance must be found between *'unacceptable variations in practice'* (DoH, 1999), expert specialist nursing opinion and the wishes and feelings of children and young people.

Finally, I would like to thank the lead authors and their colleagues for their hard work and commitment to the development of these child health nursing guidelines.

Sheila Marriott
Director of Nursing
Birmingham Children's Hospital NHS Trust
Spring 2000

References

Department of Health (1998) *A First Class Service: Quality in the New NHS*. HMSO, London

Department of Health (1999) *Making a Difference. Strengthening the nursing, midwifery and health visiting contribution to health and healthcare*. HMSO, London

Introduction: procedures for nursing intervention

Why have a procedure manual

This manual of nursing procedures has been developed for nursing staff across four key areas:
- to demonstrate current nursing practices validated by the Trust
- to give guidance to nursing staff in the implementation of nursing care
- to act as a reference point and teaching tool for students and newly appointed staff
- to provide an evidence-based framework from which care may be audited.

Purpose

To provide guidance to staff on the implementation of nursing procedures. Nursing staff are able to refer to a locally produced evidence-based document.

How will this manual support practice

The procedures have been developed by a group of nursing staff who are based in clinical practice and who have experience of implementing these nursing interventions. It is anticipated that in preparing each procedure we have developed guidelines which promote best practice. Each procedure has been researched to provide the best evidence available. In many cases evidence of research based practice is not available. Therefore it is valid that some of the procedures are not supported by any research findings. Particular practice may have evolved through a system of trial and error or had its elements based in core principles such as infection control and asepsis.

Fitness for the future

This review of the manual has been extensive and by no means indicates the maximum content of the manual. Further procedures will need to be included as practice develops. The membership of the Procedure Group is reviewed routinely to ensure a balanced representation. Wherever specialist procedures have been introduced staff have been co-opted into the group. Each procedure is reviewed annually or, more frequently, if audit or risk management issues indicate otherwise.

Designed for use

It is hoped that practitioners will find this text user friendly and recognise the attempt to highlight points of practice for consideration/discussion. The procedures have been listed alphabetically for ease of use.

Finally, this manual cannot fully explain or explore the psychological preparation that is required to prepare a child to undergo a procedure As each intervention will be different for each child we have not included specific psychological care and support for each procedure. Instead some guidance notes have been provided. These notes should influence the thinking regarding preparing children for procedures. Wherever possible, making contact with other healthcare professionals, such as play therapists and psychologists will assist and benefit nursing staff in delivering a sensitive service to the children and their families.

Preface

In order to provide the highest standards of patient/family centred care, healthcare personnel need to be aware of the *Patient's Charter (1995) Services for Children and Young People* and its implications for practice. It states that,

> *A child can expect the National Health Service to respect his/her privacy, dignity and religious and cultural beliefs.*

When dealing with children and their families, consideration must be given to how these issues can have implications for the delivery of care.

Reference

Department of Health (1995) *The Patient's Charter.* HMSO, London

Family centred care

Following the publication of the Platt Report of 1958 into the welfare of children in hospital there has been increased concern among parents, professionals and policy makers about how the experience of hospitalisation for children and their families might be made more agreeable (Darbyshire, 1994). Family centred care is advocated as the means to meeting this need. The concept of family centred care originated in the late 1980s (Ahman,1994b) and focuses on the need to deliver paediatric care in collaboration with the child and family. Paediatric nurses have since worked to develop strategies which promote this approach and have acknowledged this ideal as the *'best practice'* (Ahman, 1994b). To achieve this goal in practice, it has been identified that *'a shift from a professionally centred view to a collaborative model which recognises families are central in a child's life and their values and priorities, is central in the plan of care'* (Ahman, 1994a).

In order for family centred care to be delivered successfully it is suggested by Moules and Ramsay (1998) that there are three key issues that must be acknowledged. These are:

1. Children are admitted to hospital only if the care cannot be given at home or on a daily basis within the community or at hospital.

2. The philosophy of care needs to be clearly explained to all staff and families so that they can understand and negotiate their roles.

3. The philosophy has to be implemented in ways that take account of all the elements of family care.

Encompassed within the development of the concept of family centred care key principles have been identified, which are viewed as contributing to the promotion of modern paediatric care.

Working together

Family centred care aims to look beyond the disease orientated process to one in which the focus is on the care of the child as part of a distinct family unit. The impact on a family when a child is admitted to hospital and the resulting/additional stresses placed upon the family cannot be underestimated. The child is recognised as having *'special needs'* (DoH, 1991). Developing a family centred approach involves nurses working in partnership with parents advocating their participation as an integral factor in delivering quality care (DoH, 1991). This approach enables the child and family to maintain their strong ties while involving themselves as much as they feel able.

Parent participation has become a central theme of paediatric nursing within the UK (Coyne, 1996) and the relationship involved between the nurse and family is recognised to be complex. Fradd (1994) notes that the nurse is in a legitimate occupational role, placed to give care, while parents accompanying their child to hospital often feel displaced and uncertain of their role as parent and main caregiver. The purpose of family centred care is to bridge this gap, partnership being the vehicle advocated to meet this need.

Working together involves sharing information and Glasper (1995) asserts that giving information is the key to empowering families. Parents will often require information to be repeated or reinforced as new and unfamiliar information is not always readily recalled following periods of anxiety. Information needs to be given in a clear format that takes account of the parents' understanding and to be an ongoing part of the delivery of care. Additional written information may be required.

Partnership can be promoted through working together to plan and deliver care. This process involves the skill of negotiation on the part of the nurse to enable the child and family to be empowered to contribute fully to decisions about treatments and the ways in which they are implemented. The family's involvement should enable them to continue caring for their child in a manner that is productive and comfortable for them. Through this process of empowerment nurses can support families by encouraging them to participate in the care given and, where appropriate, to encourage self-care. Fradd (1994) attributes the success of this approach to the empowerment of the nurse, indicating that they need to feel confident in their knowledge and skills in order to share and pass these on. Fradd believes that empowering goes hand-in-hand with caring. Within this environment trust, mutual respect and open communication will exist.

Preparation for procedures

Paediatric nurses have long recognised the need for children and families to be prepared for healthcare interventions and advocate this need as a care role for the children's nurse (Brennan, 1994). This role is intricate as the paediatric nurse meets the challenge of supporting the child and family through the process while seeking to ensure a successful outcome.

Prior to any procedure being undertaken the consent of the child and/or parents is essential to maintaining both the principles of family centred care as well as meeting the legal and ethical requirements of informed consent.

Informed consent

The principle of informed consent is based on the legal and ethical requirements to provide the child and family/parents with information that will enable them to make a judgement regarding the relevance and need for the intervention. The process should include an explanation of the proposed procedure including the benefits and expected outcomes, as well as any level of risk and possible side-effects. Generally, written consent is required for any medical, surgical or diagnostic procedure undertaken by a doctor. In relation to nursing practice, the need for formal documentation is not presently practised, however the need to obtain consent is no less important although this is usually acknowledged verbally.

As nurses increasingly expand their practice to include more invasive procedures, the need to demonstrate more formally that informed consent has been granted is essential to maintaining not only legal and ethical, but also professional standards of care (Powers, 1997).

Documentation

Record keeping is recognised as being fundamental to the process of nursing and exists as a tool to demonstrate professional practice (UKCC, 1998). Since present legislation does not require nurses to complete a formal record of consent it is essential that nursing interventions and their outcomes are documented within the nursing care plan and evaluation.

Preparing a child for a procedure usually falls into two key categories, psychological and physical.

Psychological preparation

Each child will have different ways of coping with unusual situations and the possible stress incurred. The behavioural responses may differ widely from a child demonstrating no particular response to a child who responds in a manner that identifies their distress and pain as a result of a healthcare intervention. How paediatric nurses assess the degree or level of a child's coping abilities will be based on their knowledge of the child and their family and the child's level of development. The process of assessment is essential to identifying nursing care needs and negotiating the care roles of the nurse and family. Assessment initially commences upon admission to hospital and involves the collection of information regarding the child's usual activities using a systematic approach through a model of care. The nurses' knowledge of child development and growth as well as an understanding of the impact of hospitalisation to the child and family enables them to develop a comprehensive assessment, which forms the basis in designing a plan of care. This aptitude is enhanced by skills in communication and observation. Undertaking a physical assessment and record of measurements may provide additional information together with reference to assessments taken by other healthcare professionals involved in the care of children.

Preparing children for procedures decreases their anxiety, promotes their co-operation, supports their coping skills and may teach them new ones, facilitating a feeling of mastery in experiencing a potentially stressful event (Wong and Perry, 1998; Collier *et al,* 1993). Preparation may take place on an individual basis at admission, or may be undertaken during pre-admission visits.

Establishing trust between the nurse and the child and family is essential to maintaining their co-operation and support. Children rely on their parents for comfort and reassurance and wherever possible nurses need to establish whether parents wish to be present during a procedure and at what level they feel able to participate. Parents should, wherever possible, be encouraged to remain with the child, to continue their role of supporter and comforter if they and the child agree. Explaining the procedure to both the child and parent will enable them to know what to expect and support further questioning. Parents may also welcome additional advice on how they may participate or support their child during the procedure (Brennan, 1994).

The experience of undergoing an unfamiliar and unpleasant experience can result in a child becoming fearful and so increasing their level of anxiety, resulting in their reduced co-operation. Children may perceive any procedure as a punishment for being naughty or develop fantasies or distorted ideas in the absence of accurate information. The age of the child is influential in the type of information given and when it should be provided (Bates and Broome, 1986). It is generally advocated that younger children should be given a closer explanation to the actual procedure to prevent any undue fantasising and worry (Wong and Perry, 1998).

Where procedures may be unpleasant or result in some pain, these issues should be addressed honestly and explained to the child before undertaking the procedure. It may help the child if analgesia or a mild sedative is given prior to some interventions.

Hospitalisation is generally accepted as a stressful situation for children and play can be an important strategy for learning coping skills (DoH, 1991). Play can be used as a therapeutic intervention to assess a child's understanding and the use of toys and written materials can contribute to the process of coping. Many paediatric units have access to play therapists and nurses can work with them to prepare a child and their family. Play decreases fears and enables the child to feel control over events. It has been thought that play is purely an activity to occupy children. However, the literature suggests that its function is more diverse as it enables children to explore their environment and contributes to problem-solving skills (Sylvia *et al,* 1976 cited in Moules and Ramsay, 1998).

Wong (1995) has observed that most preparation strategies used by nurses are informal, focusing on providing information about the experience and are directed at stressful and painful procedures. A variety of materials can be incorporated into the care process to enable the child to express their understanding and thoughts and fears. Many children are wary of unfamiliar equipment: if possible, access to handling the equipment, if safe to do so, should be given . This activity can help to promote a sense of control during the procedure and encourage compliance.

A number of children will have had to experience frequent visits to hospital and are often perceived to be accustomed to the environment and healthcare interventions. It cannot be assumed that a child's familiarity with their surroundings will necessarily make them more co-operative. It remains relevant to maintain the access to information (Bates and Broome, 1986).

Children's reactions to strange and unusual environments may cause changes in behaviour that last well after the initial intervention is completed. Paediatric nurses should be aware of the possibility and advise parents beforehand that this change may occur and offer advice on how the child can be supported.

Physical preparation

Generally, little physical preparation is required but may include advice on restricting fluids and diet or taking prescribed medication for diagnostic examination or sedation. Some procedures will require the child to be sedated and an explanation of the issues associated with sedation should be explained to the child if they are old enough and particularly to parents to ensure the safety and well-being of the child at all times.

Planning the timing of a procedure can assist in the co-operation and compliance of the child. Wherever possible paediatric nurses should aim to incorporate nursing care into the overall daily plan of care negotiating with the child and family at each stage (Fradd, 1996).

Performance of the procedure

Preparing the environment prior to starting any intervention can reduce anxiety regarding the procedure. If possible procedures should be undertaken in a specific treatment area rather than at the child's bedspace. Areas such as the playroom are considered 'safe' and should never be used to perform any investigation or test (Whaley and Wong, 1998). It is advocated that the nurse should approach the procedure expecting a successful outcome. Any anxiety experienced by the nurse may be perceived by the child who may then become resistant and unco-operative. Involving the child and giving them choices/options works towards supporting the child (Professional File, 1992).

Positioning and holding techniques

Some nursing interventions may require the child to assume a specific position to maximise the effect of the procedure. Given their lack of understanding, infants and young children are frequently unable to co-operate and may lash out or struggle to prevent a procedure being undertaken. In order to maintain their safety and well-being paediatric nurses may have to intervene to minimise the child's movements and secure their safety through restraint (Collins, 1999). Wherever possible, children should be offered a choice of position to promote autonomy and increase their co-operation.

Concerns regarding the role of the nurse during procedures involving restraint have been recently identified (Robinson and Collier, 1997). Paediatric nurses have identified uncertainty of their legal position and noted that they have received no formal training in holding techniques. In recognition of these issues the Royal College of Nursing (1999) has recently published guidance in this area.

The autonomy of children, particularly with regard to decision-making, is gaining in stature. The report of the *Welfare of Children and Young People in Hospital* (DoH, 1991) and the acceptance of the United Nations *Convention on the Rights of the Child* (UN, 1989) have brought the issue of children's rights to the fore of modern paediatric nursing. Issues of consent have traditionally related to adults who by legal definition are over the age of 18. Persons over this age are deemed legally competent. McQuaid *et al* (1996) have commented that this notion has been perpetuated not only by medical staff and parents, but by the judicial system itself in the past. The preoccupation with parental involvement primarily within family centred care could be argued to be detrimental to fostering children's voices and choices within healthcare (Fulton, 1996). Children are traditionally thought of as being inexperienced in matters concerning their welfare and, as such, unable to understand and evaluate complex medical information (Alderson, 1993). The case of Gillick *vs* Wisbech demonstrates that measuring a child or young person's ability to make decisions does not rest solely on their chronological age, but also on their level of development and the experiences they have been exposed to. Fulton (1996) proposes that maybe nurses should develop an approach which presumes children are competent unless demonstrated otherwise by the adult.

As our understanding of the rights of the child develops nurses need to consider the issues surrounding restraint. This is a complex area, closely governed by the guiding principles of the Children's Act (DoH, 1989). Increasingly, both children and healthcare professionals recognise that children have choices about what treatments they may consent to or refuse.

It is generally accepted that parents/carers are the key factor to supporting their child, encouraging co-operation between the child and nurse and in helping them deal/manage the many sensations involved. Nurses will frequently ask parents to assist them during the procedure by employing distraction techniques, such as playing with toys and talking with the child, so minimising the distress to the child and maximising the effect of the nursing intervention.

References

Ahman E (1994a) Family centred care: shifting orientation. *Pediatric Nursing* March/April **20**(2):113–7, 132–3

Ahman E (1994b) Family centred care: the time has come. *Pediatric Nursing* January **20**(1): 52–3

Audit Commission (1993) *Children First: A study of hospital services.* HMSO, London

Bates T, Broome M (1986) Preparation of children for hospital and surgery: A review of the literature. *Journal of Pediatric Nursing* **1**(4): 230–9

Brennan A (1994) Caring for children during procedures: A review of the literature. *Pediatric Nursing* Sept/Oct **20**(5): 451–8

Collier J *et al* (1993) Painful procedures: Preparation and coping strategies for children. *Maternal and Child Health* **18**(9): 282–6

Collins P (1999) Restraining children for painful procedures. *Paediatric Nursing.* April **11**(3): 14–16

Coyne IT (1996) Parent participation: a concept analysis. *Journal of Advanced Nursing* April **23**(4): 733– 40

Darbyshire P (1994) *Living with a Sick Child in Hospital: The experiences of parents and nurses.* Chapman and Hall, London

Darbyshire P (1995) Family centred care within contemporary British paediatric nursing. *British Journal of Nursing* January **4**: 31–3

Department of Health (1989) *The Children's Act.* HMSO, London

Department of Health (1991) *Welfare of Children and Young People in Hospital.* HMSO, London

Douglas C (1997) The stresses of parenthood. *Community Nurse* September **3**(8): 63

Fradd E (1994) Power to the people. *Paediatric Nursing* April **6**(3): 11–14

Fradd E (1996) The importance of negotiating a care plan. *Paediatric Nursing* July **8**(6): 6–8

Fulton Y (1996) Children's rights and the role of the nurse. *Paediatric Nursing* **8**(10): 29–31

Gillick vs Wisbech and West Norfolk Health Authority [1984] A11 ER635

Glasper EA (1995) Preserving children's nursing within a climate of genericism. *British Journal of Nursing* January **4**: 24–5

McQuaid L, Huband S, Parker E (1996) *Children's Nursing.* Churchill Livingstone, London

Ministry of Health (1959) *The Welfare of Children in Hospital. Report of the Committee on Child Health Services.* (Platt Report) HMSO, London

Moules T, Ramsay J (1998) *The Textbook of Children's Nursing.* Stanley Thornes (Publishing) Ltd, Cheltenham

Power KJ (1997) The legal and ethical implications of consent to nursing procedures. *British Journal of Nursing* August **6**(15): 885– 8

Professional File (1992) Help for children undergoing painful procedures. *Professional Nurse* March **7**(6): 346–7

Robinson S, Collier J (1997) Holding children still for procedures. *Paediatric Nursing* **9**(4): 12–14

Royal College of Nursing (1999) *Restraining, Holding Still and Containing Children: Guidelines for Good Practice*. RCN, London

United Kingdom Central Council for Nursing, Midwifery and Health Visiting (1998) *Guidelines forRecords and Record Keeping*. UKCC, London

United Nations (1989) *Convention on the Rights of the Child*. UN, New York

Wong DL (1995) *Nursing Care of Infants and Children.* 5th edn. Mosby, St Louis

Wong DL, Perry SE (1998) *Maternal Child Nursing*. Mosby, St Louis

Clinical procedures for nursing interventions

Ayliffe Taylor handwash technique

Definition: A method of cleansing the hands

Purpose: To remove transient or resident micro-organisms. The technique for undertaking a handwash, whether as a 'social' or 'aseptic' action is the same. However, the products used may vary given the nature of the procedure.

Equipment required

- Hand bowl
- Disposable paper towels
- Cleansing lotion dispenser
- Hot water supply with taps operated from the elbow
- Access to foot operated bin.

Nursing observations

- Personal condition of hands.

Nursing interventions

- Remove all jewellery, eg. watches or stoned rings
- Wet hands thoroughly under running water and apply 5mls of soap/disinfectant
- Refer to *Figure 2.1* – wash hands as follows:
  - Rub palm to palm (five times)
  - Rub right palm over left of dorsum and left palm over right dorsum (nine times)
  - Rub palm to palm with fingers interlaced (five times)
  - Rub backs of fingers to opposing palms with finger interlocked (five times)
  - Clasp right thumb in the left hand and rub rotationally and vice versa
  - Clasp right hand fingers and rub rotationally backwards and forwards in left palm and vice versa
- Rinse hands under running water, holding hands down
- Dry hands thoroughly using paper towels
- Where only a hand-operated tap is available, a paper towel can be used to turn off the water supply
- Discard towels in wastebin using foot operated lever
- If washbasins are not available or it is impractical to return to a washbasin, an alcohol hand rub can be applied to clean hands using the above technique.

Figure 2.1: Ayliffe Taylor handwash technique

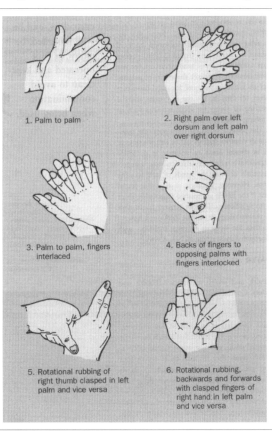

1. Palm to palm

2. Right palm over left dorsum and left palm over right dorsum

3. Palm to palm, fingers interlaced

4. Backs of fingers to opposing palms with fingers interlocked

5. Rotational rubbing of right thumb clasped in left palm and vice versa

6. Rotational rubbing, backwards and forwards with clasped fingers of right hand in left palm and vice versa

Safety issues

The use of an alcohol rub is acceptable. However, all areas of the hand must be disinfected and the alcohol must have dried/evaporated before commencing a procedure.

Further reading

Ayliffe GA, Collins BJ, Taylor LJ (1982) *Hospital Acquired Infection*. Wright and Son, Bristol

Larson LE (1978) APIC Guidelines for infection control practice. *American Journal for Infection Control* **23**(4): 251–69

Millwood S, Barnett J, Tomlinson D (1993) A clinical infection control audit programme: evaluation of an audit tool used by infection control nurses to monitor standards and assess effective staff training. *Journal of Hospital Infection* **24**: 219–23

Taylor LJ (1978) An evaluation of hand washing technique (Parts 1&2). *Nursing Times* **74**: 54–5, 108–10

See *Appendix III*

Nursing notes

Anal dilation

Definition: A method of stretching the anus using a metal probe/hagar dilator

Purpose: To dilate a narrow or newly created anus, to enable the child to pass faecal motions without discomfort.

Equipment required

- Lubricating jelly
- Correct size dilator
- Paper tissues
- Protective undersheet/nappy
- Apron and gloves.

Psychological preparation and support

- This procedure is intrusive in nature and detailed explanations regarding the process should be given to ensure child/parental consent
- Explain procedure relative to child's age and cognitive development, involving parents where possible
- Acknowledge that child may be reluctant or fearful of the procedure, particularly if it is likely to cause some discomfort or pain
- Involve the play specialist in the preparation of the child for procedure.

Nursing observations

- If appropriate, record baseline observations of pulse, blood pressure and respiratory rate
- This procedure is potentially distressing. It is important to observe the child's level of anxiety and behaviour during and after dilation, giving repeated support and reassurance
- Observe anal area prior to commencing procedure. Note integrity of surrounding skin
- Following dilation, observe child's ability to defecate comfortably, noting the size and type of stool passed
- Observe for evidence of rectal bleeding following procedure and record in nursing notes. Inform medical staff if bleeding does not stop spontaneously.

Nursing interventions

- Position infant/child on their back with protective sheet underneath
- Lubricate the first inch of dilator with lubricating jelly
- Raise the infant's/child's legs upwards, flexing at the knees towards the abdomen
- Gently insert dilator and gradually rotate the dilator a quarter turn, ie. 90°
- Rotate dilator back 90° and slowly withdraw dilator
- Wipe any surplus lubricating jelly from around anal area
- Reposition infant/child and give comfort and reassurance
- Remove disposable equipment
- Following patient use, rinse and return equipment to CSSD for re-sterilising
- Wash hands using Ayliffe Taylor method.

Safety issues

- The first anal dilation should be performed by medical staff and they should indicate:
  - the size of dilator
  - frequency of dilations
  - distance dilator is to be inserted (usually between ½–1 inch). This depends on a child's anatomy, ie. size of stenosis or anastomosis.

Adaptation for home care

- Procedure remains the same.

Further reading

Clayden G (1991) Managing the child with constipation. *Professional Care of Mother and Child* **1**(2): 64–6

Oldhamet Columbani PM, Foglia RP (1997) *Surgery of Infants and Children.* Lippincott-Rowe, London: 1323–62

See *Appendix III*

Nursing notes

Application of skin traction

Definition: Traction is the application of a pulling force to a limb or part of the body

Purpose: Applying the skin traction can:
- prevent or reduce muscle spasm
- immobilise a joint/limb/fracture
- reduce pain.

Equipment required

- Bed
- Fracture frame
- Weights and weight holder. NB. Amount of weight should be specified by medical staff in figures and words
- Traction kit
- Crepe bandages
- Tape
- Cord
- Adhesive/non-adhesive skin extensions
- Barrier lotion/cream
- Prescription chart
- Medication.

Psychological preparation and support

- Assess age and developmental level of child
- Assess family's understanding of the procedure in order to reduce anxiety and facilitate co-operation
- Consider whether the use of analgesia/muscle relaxants may be beneficial prior to commencing procedure.

Nursing observations

- Prior to commencing application of skin traction, record observations of circulation, sensation and movement of limb distal to fracture in order to assess suitability for traction
- Supporting the limb, place skin extension against skin, ensuring foam pads cover medial and lateral malleolus, while crepe bandage is applied by nurse from ankle to thigh using a 'figure of eight' technique ensuring no creases appear in skin extension
- Ensure skin is clean and dry at all times. Take down bandages daily to inspect for signs of excess pressure or skin breakdown, taking care to maintain traction
- Assess skin condition daily observing for bruising or broken areas
- Inspect skin extensions daily for evidence of creases and that the foam pads are giving protection to bony prominences
- Inspect adhesive skin extensions for signs of oozing and local heat
- Ensure that skin surrounding the groin and buttocks is thoroughly cleansed to prevent soiling of skin extensions. Explain to family and carers the importance of thorough and more frequent cleansing

- Observe circulation, sensation and movement of limb distal to fracture site:
  - half-hourly for two hours
  - hourly for 12 hours
  - two-hourly for 24 hours
  - four-hourly thereafter.

Nursing interventions

- Administer sedative prior to undertaking procedure
- Ascertain child's allergy status to ensure appropriate traction kit selected
- Two nursing staff should perform this procedure
- Apply manual traction distal to the fracture site.

Non-adhesive traction

- Hold foam extension set away from sole of foot. Allowing room for movement of foot, measure outer aspect of limb to level of gluteal fold and allow two-inch turnover. Measure inner aspect of limb to mid thigh and allow two-inch turnover
- Secure end of bandage in place with tape
- Estimate the middle of cord and tie a reef knot at the base of the cushion pad
- Thread single/double cord through the pulley and attach weights using a slipknot, ensuring the weights are supported at this time
- Gradually release weights and allow to hang freely
- Elevate foot or bed to provide counter traction
- Remove and reapply skin traction daily (taking care to maintain manual traction) to monitor skin integrity and ensure effective traction.

Adhesive traction

- Measure and cut extensions to correct length, ensuring room for full foot movement. Spray inner and outer aspect of limb with Op-site or other suitable barrier lotion
- Apply skin extensions to outer and inner aspects. Make small cuts to strapping as necessary to prevent creases forming
- Round the ends of extension tapes to prevent tape peeling away from skin
- Apply crepe bandages with over skin extension from a thigh (ensuring leg is in a neutral position using a 'figure of eight' technique)
- Secure bandages with tape
- Estimate the middle of the cord and tie a reef knot at the base of the cushion pad
- Thread cord through pulley and attach weights using a slipknot, ensuring weights are supported
- Gradually release weights and allow to hang freely
- Elevate foot off the bed to provide counter traction
- Remove bandage daily to monitor skin integrity.

Best practice
- ❖ Administer analgesia routinely prior to changing bandage.

Safety issues

- Ensure protruding pole ends (if used) are covered with padding to prevent injury to other children, visitors or staff
- Ensure weights hang freely without obstruction; jarring of weights will lead to increased discomfort and pain for child. Ensure other children or visitors do not interfere with weights
- Ensure pulley system is secured well to the end of the bed to prevent slippage of the traction system
- If the child is allergic to Elastoplast use non-adhesive extension tape. Protect skin with gauze.

Further reading

Wieck L, King E, Dyer M (1986) *Illustrated Manual of Nursing Techniques.* 3rd edn. JB Lippincott and Company, London: 667–70

Heywood Jones I (1990) Making sense of traction. *Nursing Times* 6 June **86**(23): 39–41

Davis P (1989) Principles of traction. *Nursing (Journal of Clinical Practice, Education and Management)* February **3**(34): 5–8

See *Appendix III*

Nursing notes

Barrier nursing — standard/strict (source isolation)

Definition: The isolation of a child who has an infection which could be harmful or hazardous to others

Purpose: This procedure is designed to prevent the transfer of pathogenic micro-organisms from infected children to other patients or staff.

This procedure must be read in conjunction with the Trust's Isolation Policy

Categories of isolation (for specific categories see *Appendix II*)

Standard

- Respiratory
- Excretion/secretion
- Skin/wound.

Strict

- Required for certain highly infectious or dangerous diseases. A list of source isolation categories can be found in *Appendix II.*

Equipment required

- Single rooms normally require hand washing facilities but in some cases this may not be necessary:
  - *Respiratory isolation*: A single room is required for protection from infection that is spread by the respiratory route (droplets). The door **must** be kept closed
  - *Excretion/secretion/blood isolation:* Unless actually bleeding, most children can be nursed successfully on main ward
  - *Enteric isolation:* A single room is preferred, but is less important for infants confined to their own cot
  - *Skin/wound isolation:* A single room is usually required. The door **must** be kept closed
- White Isolation Card — displayed on door or on end of bed if used in open ward.

Outside the cubicle

- Trolley/table
- Plastic apron
- Disposable gloves
- Alcohol hand rub.

NB. Specific advice regarding the use of protective clothing can be found in the Trust's Isolation Policy.

Inside the cubicle

- Appropriate rubbish/linen bags
- Sharps container.

NB. Not all linen from isolated patients needs to be disposed of as 'infected'. Refer to trust policy for the handling of used linen.

Nursing observations

- Physical/social isolation of child and carers/family
- Ensure sufficient information and progress given as an ongoing process.

Nursing interventions

- Ensure isolation notices are clearly displayed
- Seek advice from Infection Control Team if other children demonstrate similar symptoms
- Explain to the family and child the importance of thorough hand washing prior to entering and before leaving the room
- Ensure child's personal belongings remain in room at all times
- Dispose of rubbish, linen, and clinical waste according to the Trust Infection Control Policy
- Ensure thorough hand washing and wearing of apron and gloves prior to entering room
- Ensure door is closed at all times
- Remove apron and gloves before leaving room
- Supervise daily cleaning of room according to the Trust Infection Control Policy.

Strict isolation
- Children/adolescents with a highly contagious infection will be transferred to a special unit
- The Infection Control Team must be informed immediately
- Further specific details can be found in the Trust Infection Control Policy.

Safety issues

- If child is required to leave the unit, relevant information regarding isolation procedures should be forwarded to the appropriate Head of Department prior to transfer.

Further reading

Spears R, Shooter RA, Gaya H *et al* (1969) Contamination of nurses uniforms with Staphylococcus aureus. *Lancet* **III**: 233–5

Hambraeus A (1973) Transfer of Staphylococcus aureus via nurses uniforms. *T Hyg* (Camb) **71**: 799–814

Department of Health, PHLS (1995) *Hospital Infection Control: Evidence on the Control of Infection in Hospitals.* Prepared by the working group of the DOH and PHLS: March

Infection Control Standards Working Party (1993) *Standards in Infection Control in Hospitals.* Prepared by the Infection Control Standards Working Party, AMM HIS ICNA PHCS

Department of Health (1974) *Health and Safety at Work Act 1974.* HMSO, London

General COSHH ACOP and CARCINOGENS ACOP and BIOLOGICAL AGENTS ACOP Control of Substances Hazardous to Health Regulations 1994. H.S.E.

Birmingham Children's Hospital Infection Control Policies:

- Policy for the Care and Maintenance of Toys
- Isolation Policy
- Notes on individual infectious diseases
- Disinfecting Policy
- Universal Precautions
- Transportation and labelling of specimen
- Disposal of Clinical Waste Policy

See *Appendix III*

Nursing notes

Bathing an infant/child

Definition: Cleansing of the body

Purpose: To maintain hygiene and promote comfort.

Equipment required

- Baby bath, bowl or bath
- Soap or bubble bath
- Skin treatment, ie. Oilatum/Balneum (as required)
- Shampoo and conditioner
- Flannel (two), sponge, cotton wool and gauze
- Towels
- Baby lotion, skin treatments, ie. emollients, moisturisers.

Psychological preparation and support

- Some older children and teenagers can take responsibility for caring for their own hygiene needs. However, some children may be reluctant and need encouragement while others may need constant supervision
- Where possible involve parents in performing or assisting with hygiene needs
- Being washed by someone else can be embarrassing — ensure privacy and dignity is maintained.

Nursing observations

- While bathing, observe the state of the skin for rashes, bruising, presence of dry patches and pressure area appearance
- Observe for abnormalities, ie. decreased/increased muscle tone during handling of small infant/child
- Pay attention to areas such as skin folds in the genital area where a build up of smegma can occur — older children may need reminding to cleanse these areas.

Nursing interventions

- Assess if bath, bed bath or help with wash is required — depending on the child's mobility and any limitations
- Prepare all equipment prior to procedure to prevent prolonged exposure
- Ensure bathroom or bed area is warm and free from direct drafts
- Maintain privacy
- Bathing when children have a skin condition or following surgery can be very uncomfortable
- Administer analgesic prior to bath and use toys to distract and reduce any possible discomfort
- Fill bath, bowl, checking the temperature of the water.

Baby bath

- Remove clothing and wrap the baby in a towel, wash their face using gauze or a soft flannel and dry thoroughly
- Remove clothing and nappy
- Wash trunk and limbs leaving genital area to last
- Remove from bath and dry thoroughly
- Use moisturisers or prescribed skin treatments
- Apply clean nappy and dress
- Clear area.

Bath

- Undress child, assist into the bath, being aware of dressings
- Wash the face using a flannel or sponge
- Using separate flannel, wash trunk, limbs and genital area
- Allow time for play
- Remove from bath and dry thoroughly
- Apply moisturisers or any prescribed skin treatments
- Dress
- Clear the area
- For bed bathing follow the same cleansing procedure, however uncover one area at a time, clean and dry it and recover before cleansing another area so as to maintain warmth and dignity
- For larger children or a dependant child, two nurses may be necessary.

Safety issues

- Check the temperature of the water, it should be 36°C/96°F
- Never leave small children and infants alone in the bath
- Check the depth of the water (10cm, 4 inches is adequate)
- Take extra care when additives are used in the water — they can make the bath and surrounding area slippy
- Keep dressings, cannulas dry
- Disconnect all electrical equipment, ie. saturation probes, to prevent electrocution
- Lifting and use of bath aids — refer to Trust Manual Handling policy.

Adaptation for home care

- The same procedure should be followed
- Lifting and bath aids are available via Occupational Therapists.

Discussion points

❖ When cleansing an infant's face, gauze is preferable to cotton wool for the eye area, as cotton fibres can harm the surface of the eyes.

❖ It is recommended to avoid using talcum powder as the fine mist of powder may be inhaled and if used repeatedly may cause respiratory problems.

❖ Note that children from minority ethnic groups will have additional needs in terms of the additional skin/hair care required to maintain their personal hygiene. Liaise with child's parents to ensure that these needs are met.

Further reading

Whaley L, Wong DL (1993) *Essentials of Paediatric Nursing.* 4th edn. Mosby, St Louis

See *Appendix III*

Nursing notes

Blood administration

Definition: The administration of blood via an intravenous infusion

Purpose: To return haemoglobin levels to within normal limits.

Equipment required

- IV fluid chart
- IV giving set
- Blood filter
- IV pump
- Observation chart.

Nursing observations

- During transfusion undertake recordings of temperature and blood pressure half-hourly for first hour, then hourly until transfusion is completed.

Nursing interventions

Prior to transfusion

- Units of blood must only be taken to the ward when they are required for transfusion (Tx)
- An intravenous prescription form must be completed by the authorising doctor prior to the beginning of the transfusion, giving details of the type of blood product, total volume to be given and the rate of transfusion. Any additional instructions, eg. use of blood warmer, antihistamine cover, should also be stated on this form.

Setting up transfusion

- The unit of blood should be fully checked by a registered paediatric nurse and one other member of the nursing team. In checking each unit of blood the following procedure should always be followed:
  - Identification of the patient and the information from the following areas should be compared:
    - patient's identification bracelet
    - the compatibility report
    - the compatibility label on the unit of blood
  - The ABC group and the Rhesus type of the blood should be checked against the blood group report on the request and with the compatibility label on the unit of blood
  - Always examine the appearance of the unit of blood prior to administration for evidence of discolouration or Haemolysis. Examine the bag for leaks by squeezing firmly
  - Check that the expiry date on the unit of blood has not been exceeded at the time of transfusion.

Only if the above details are correct should the unit be transfused. The giving set can be primed with normal saline (0.9% sodium chloride). Each unit of blood transfused should be recorded on the Intravenous Administration chart, which states:

- Patient identification details
- The day and time at which the unit was administered to the patient
- Signature of the person checking and commencing the infusion.

After transfusion the plastic pack which contained the unit of blood should be sealed and kept for 24 hours, initially in the clinical area and thereafter discarded appropriately in clinical waste.

Blood transfusion reactions

❖ If a patient has a transfusion reaction the doctor responsible for that patient should be informed immediately and the transfusion stopped while this is done. The decision whether or not to continue with the transfusion must be made by the medical staff.

See *Appendix III*

Nursing notes

Blood pressure, the taking and recording of

Definition: Measurement of child's haemodynamic parameters

Purpose: To establish the effectiveness of child's circulatory system.

Equipment required

For oscillometric method

- Dinamap

For manual method

- Sphygmomanometer
- Stethoscope

For both

- Cuff of correct size
- Toys, games, appropriate to age
- Observation chart.

Psychological preparation and support

Infancy: 3 months to 1 year

- Involve parents
- Older infants may demonstrate resistance to procedure.

Toddler: 1–3 years

- Explain how the cuff will feel when the blood pressure is being obtained. Tight feeling will go away
- Ask them to try to keep their arm still
- The child may demonstrate reluctance/resistance to procedure
- Use distraction techniques
- If necessary involve play department, as appropriate for age.

Pre-school child: 3–5 years

- Explain procedure in simple terms
- Allow the child to play with the dinamap/start dinamap
- Point on a doll to where the cuff is placed
- Praise the child for helping, never shame for lack of co-operation.

School aged children: 5–11 years

- Explain the procedure with reasons
- Allow the child to start the dinamap
- Give time for questions and answers.

Adolescent: 11–17 years

- Explain why the procedure is necessary
- Encourage questioning
- Involve in decision-making, eg. which arm to place the cuff on.

Nursing observations

For oscillometric method

- Ensure that the dinamap is charged or plugged into, ensure an accurate result

- The dinamap should be calibrated every six months to ensure that accurate readings are obtained.

For manual method

- Ensure that equipment and hoses are in good repair to obtain accurate results.

For both

- Ensure that cuffs are in good condition.

Nursing interventions

- Encourage the child in the clinic/ward environment to relax before the recordings are made, as abnormally high recordings can be obtained through child's anxiety
- Ensure that the arm or leg is fully exposed so that recordings are not affected, keep the upper arm supported at heart level
- Select a cuff that covers two-thirds of the upper arm, (if a child under one year the same size cuff may be used on the leg)
- When the leg is used as a baseline recording, a blood pressure on the arm and leg should be performed to ensure that there are no discrepancies
- Ensure that the hoses are hanging over the brachial artery on the arm and the posterior tibia on the ankle
- Record on the observation chart, the site/location where the blood pressure has been recorded, ie. from the arm or leg (over one year of age the systolic may be higher when recorded on the leg)
- For manual method, place the stethoscope over the artery site, palpate brachial artery and inflate cuff 20 mmHg above the last pulse beat heard. Deflate cuff slowly noting the level at which two consecutive beats are first heard, this is the systolic reading. Continue to deflate and note when the sound disappears, this is the diastolic reading
- If rechecking a blood pressure, allow one to two minutes for venous emptying
- If the child is distressed allow longer waiting time for them to settle, resulting in a more accurate reading
- The younger the child the higher the risk of incorrect readings. Performing a manual blood pressure on an infant has a higher error rate, due to the pulse being difficult to hear and the possible distress of the child.

Safety issues

- Ensure that the blood pressure cuff is used, as per manufacturer instructions, eg. white neonatal cuffs are for single patient use only
- If a cuff has been used on an infected patient then they should be discarded as they are capable of transmitting infection and there is no reliable method of cleaning them
- In the Critikon manual it is noted that prolonged continuous use of a blood pressure monitor has been associated with ischaemia and neuropathy. In view of this the cuff should be removed from the child's limb when it is not in use
- Always ensure that the skin is intact prior to placing the cuff on the skin. It is advisable not to place the cuff on the same arm as a cannulae as it will contribute to extravasation.

Adaptation for home care

- As for oscillometric method already described.

Discussion points

❖ If a child exhibits vastly different blood pressure readings on different limbs, eg. alternate arms, then it may be due to cardiac abnormalities.

❖ Although it as has already been mentioned, over one year of age systolic readings on lower limbs tend to be considerably higher.

Further reading

Axton S, Bertrand S, Smith L, Dy E, Lichr P (1995) Comparison of brachial and calf blood pressures in infants. *Paediatric Nursing* July/August **21**(4): 323–5

Campbell S, Glasper E (1995) *Whaley and Wong's Children's Nursing.* Mosby, St Louis

Courts S (1996) Monitoring blood pressure in children. *Paediatric Nursing* **8**(7): 25–27

Critikon Dinamap Operation Manual (1997) For further information refer to Johnson and Johnson Medical Ltd, Ascot, Berkshire

Hinchliff S, Montague S (1988) *Physiology for Nursing Practice.* Ballière Tindall, London

Jacoby A, Fixler D, Torres E (1993) Limitations of an oscillometric ambulatory blood pressure monitor in physically active children. *The Journal of Paediatrics* February: 231–6

Nicholson W, Matthews J, Sullivan J, Wren C (1993) Ambulatory blood pressure monitoring. *Archives of Disease in Childhood* **69**: 681–4

Portman R, Yetman R, West S (1991) Efficacy of 24-hour ambulatory blood pressure monitoring in children. *The Journal of Paediatrics* June: 842–9

Torrance C, Semple M (1997) Blood pressure measurement procedure. *Nursing Times* **93**(40): suppl 1–2

See *Appendix III*

Nursing notes

Blood products collection

Definition: To obtain prescribed blood products from Blood Bank and transfer to patient for infusion

Purpose: To ensure correct administration of blood products as prescribed.

Equipment required

- Prescription chart
- Patient details
- Blood identification form (see *Figure 2.2*).

Nursing interventions

- Registered nurses or students may collect the blood if they have relevant knowledge or previous experience
- With completed blood identification form proceed to Blood Bank
- If out of hours, ensure you are able to gain access
- Locate patient blood form (top copy) in folder in Blood Bank and also the ward's copy, which is stored under the name of the ward

Figure 2. 2: Blood identification form

> The Birmingham Children's Hospital NHS Trust
> **Blood Transfusion Department**
> **TO THE BLOOD BANK**
> Please supply compatible blood for the following patient:
>
> Surname (BLOCK CAPITALS) _____
>
> Christian names _____
>
> Registration Number _____
> Date of Birth _____
> Ward/Theatre _____
>
> Signed _____
>
> **Blood cannot be issued except on presentation of this form**
> **with ALL particulars completed**

- Check white form identification details against details on blood form (bottom copy) before removing blood from fridge
- Check special instructions on form (ie. filter, cold antibodies)
- Open the fridge, locate unit of blood required and remove from fridge (alarm will sound when fridge opened, this will stop when fridge is closed)
- Units should be taken from the fridge singly and in the order on the request form
- The date and time of removal and signature of person must be entered against the appropriate pack number on the top copy of the request form. File the identification form at collection point
- If this unit is subsequently not used and returned to Blood Bank, the date and time of return must be entered on the request form and the person returning the blood must sign the form. Put blood back in fridge
- Blood should be collected half an hour prior to the administration.

Safety issues

- British law requires that every unit of blood or blood product must be fully traceable from the donation to the patient who receives the transfusion, and that the patient's notes must contain the relevant details of the blood or blood product.

See *Appendix III*

Bolus feeding

Definition: Bolus feeding is a method of feeding via a nasogastric or gastrostomy tube where a required volume of feed is given intermittently. **NB. Bolus feeding is not suitable for jejunostomy feeding**

Purpose: To ensure safe delivery of feed into the stomach over 20–30 minutes.

Equipment required

- Yellow apron (in accordance with food hygiene regulations)
- Non sterile gloves
- Gravity feed system/integral clamp
- Blue litmus paper/pH paper
- Sterile gallipot x two
- 10ml/50ml syringe as appropriate
- Sterile water
- Feed (room temperature).

Psychological preparation and support

- Discuss the reasons for bolus feeding with child/family/carer
- Explain the procedure to child/family to facilitate psychological preparation and co-operation
- Assess children and parents understanding of why tube feeding is required.

Nursing observations

- Ensure child's weight is accurately recorded daily or as requested by medical and dietetic staff. NB. All children and babies should have routine monitoring of height, weight and head circumference if the child is under two years of age
- If child develops diarrhoea inform medical/dietetic staff
- Specimens will need to be sent to Microbiology for culture and sensitivity
- Liquid part of stool will need to be sent to Clinical Chemistry for testing of Reducing Substances
- If child develops profuse vomiting, stop feeding and inform dietetic and medical staff. Observe child for any signs of aspiration.

Nursing interventions

- Wash hands thoroughly using Ayliffe Taylor method
- Put on yellow apron
- Clean working surface area and wipe over with alcohol swabs and allow to dry
- Collect all feed and equipment
- Check feed and expiry date
- Clean tops of feed cans using alcohol impregnated wipes
- Wash can opener, wipe with alcohol impregnated wipe
- Open gravity feed pack and all equipment
- Wash hands using Ayliffe Taylor method. Put on disposable gloves
- Check position of tube
- Aspirate tube and test that blue litmus paper (alkaline) turns pink (acid) pH (use a 50ml syringe if a silk tube is in situ)
- With a minimal amount of sterile water, flush tube clear prior to feeding

- Ensure patient is comfortable, ideally sitting upright or nursed at a 30° angle
- Apply clamp to gravity feed tube (integral clamp is available with some sets)
- Check feed is given at room temperature
- Prime tube by pouring feed into reservoir ensuring that the inside of reservoir remains sterile
- Release clamps slowly and run feed to end of tubing. If necessary, run minimal excess feed into sterile pot
- Attach gravity feed tube to child's feeding tube. Ensuring tube is clean
- Slowly release clamp and elevate the gravity feed back above the level of the child's stomach
- Raising the set increases the flow rate and lowering the set slows the flow rate
- Administer the feed over 20–30 minutes
- On completion of feed, flush the gravity feed set with minimal amount of sterile water and allow this to drain into child's tube
- Disconnect gravity feed pack from patient's feeding tube and replace cap on patient's feeding tube. Clean feed pack and sterilise in cold sterilising solution for up to 24 hours
- If possible keep child/baby in upright or 30° angle for at least 30 minutes after feeding.

Safety issues/possible complications

- **Aspiration of feed**

  Stop feed immediately. Observe all vital signs and inform medical staff. If necessary use suction and prepare for resuscitation.

- **Feeding tube is not correctly positioned**

  Do not commence feeding until you are satisfied the nasogastric tube is placed correctly.

- **Feed delivered too quickly**

  Lower gravity feed reservoir to decrease rate of feed. Observe rate of feed. Observe child for increased respiratory rate and signs of abdominal discomfort.

- **Child's colour deteriorates during feed administration**

  Stop feeding immediately. Ensure airway is clear, check tube position. Contact medical staff immediately.

- **Vomiting during feed administration**

  Stop feed immediately. Observe child carefully for signs of aspiration. Inform medical/dietetic staff.

See *Appendix I* for further guidance on tube placement.

Adaptation for home care

- Procedure is the same as above. Senior nurses prior to discharge must teach parents/carers. Written information re: bolus feeding should be given to parents and community nurse teams contacted to plan discharge. A ten-day supply of equipment will be supplied to parents in the first instance and equipment needs should be discussed with community staff prior to discharge

  NB. Cooled boiled water can be used in the community for flushing

- Wash gravity feed system in hot soapy water and rinse thoroughly
- Soak gravity feed system in hypochorite sterilising solution. Change gravity feed system every 24 hours.

Best practice

❖ Although tube feeding is not the same as eating, try to make the situation as normal as possible, eg. sitting child in a chair or on your lap. If possible, let child/baby have something in their mouth to taste/suck while they are tube fed to associate the sight, taste and smell of feed with satisfaction of hunger.

Further reading

Anderton A, Aidoo KE (1988) The effect of handling procedures on microbial contamination of enteral feeds. *Journal of Hospital Infection* **II** : 364–72

Davis A (1994) Indications and techniques for enteral feeds. In: Baker SB, Baker RD, Davis A (eds) (1994) *Paediatric Enteral Nutrition.* Chapman and Hall, London

Elia ME, Cottee S, Holden CE *et al* (1995) *Enteral and Parenteral Nutritioning.* The Community British Association for Parenteral and Enteral Nutrition, Maidenhead

Holden CE, Sexton E, Paul L (1997) Enteral nutrition. *Paediatric Nursing* **8**(5): 28–35

Metheny N, Reed L, Wiersema L, McSweaney M, Wehrle MA, Clark J (1993) Effectiveness of pH measurements on predicting feeding tube placement: An update. *Nursing Research* **42**(6): 324–31

South Birmingham Authority (1992) *Food Hygiene and Code of Practice.* South Birmingham Authority: May

Taylor S, Goodison-McLaren S (1994) *Nutritional Support: A team approach.* Wolfe Publishing Ltd, London

Tuchman DN (1994) Oropharyngeal and Esophageal complications of enteral tube feeding. In: Baker SB, Baker RD, Davis A (eds) (1994) *Paediatric Enteral Nutrition.* Chapman and Hall, London

See *Appendix III*

Nursing notes

Catheter sample of urine

Definition: The collection of a catheter sample of urine, for the purpose of investigation

Purpose: To obtain an uncontaminated sample of urine.

NB. As little as 2ml of urine may be sufficient for culture, 0.5ml for urine electrolytes. For more extensive clinical chemistry 10ml is required.

Equipment required

- Alcohol wipes
- Syringe, large enough for sample volume required, if needed
- Small gauge needle, if needed
- Universal specimen pot. This may need to include preservative if the sample is to be cultured but not sent to the laboratory immediately
- Request form
- Non-sterile gloves
- Tray or receiver
- Plastic apron.

Psychological preparation and support

- This method of urine collection is not directly invasive to the child, but information suitable to the age of child and involvement of parents is important to reduce anxiety.

Nursing observations

- Check that the sample is collected at the requested time (an early morning sample may be required)
- Observe the patency of the catheter (ie. that it is draining down the tube)
- Assess the genital area for signs of infection or soreness. Ensure that catheter care is performed daily or more frequently if required
- Note if the child experiences any pain or discomfort
- Observe the urine for any cloudiness or colour irregularity. Colour changes may be due to concentrated urine, or presence of blood or bilirubin. Cloudy urine may be due to urine infection or presence of protein
- Ward test urine if indicated or if not done previously. Take care to maintain asepsis.

Nursing interventions

- Explain procedure to parents and child
- Check identity of child against the request form
- Label universal container with child's name, registration number and ward
- Ensure privacy
- Wash hands using Ayliffe Taylor method
- Note date and time of sample collection on request form and specimen pot
- Include details of method of collection of urine sample, ie. catheter sample of urine (CSU)
- Identify the sample collection area — this is either a rubber-coated strip fairly high up the tubing (in order to collect a recent sample), or a drainage point in a small chamber attached to the catheter bag.

Procedure for collecting sample from chamber with drainage point
- Ensure that the chamber has recently been drained into the main bag so that sample collected is fresh
- Wearing gloves, cleanse sample point with alcohol wipe and allow this to evaporate and dry
- Place open universal pot under the chamber and open the valve to drain the urine sample. Close valve and replace cap on sample. Ensure drainage point is dry and secure. Remove gloves and wash hands using Ayliffe Taylor method.

Procedure for collecting sample from catheter tubing
- Wearing gloves, cleanse the rubber area with alcohol wipe and allow this to dry
- Attach needle to syringe and carefully insert into the tubing through the rubber area, securing the tube with free hand while avoiding positioning in direction of needle
- Slowly draw back sample of urine into syringe. Remove needle and place into receiver. Transfer sample into specimen pot and secure lid
- Ensure sample site is not leaking urine and is dry
- Safely dispose of needle and syringe
- Remove gloves and wash hands.

For both procedures
- Ensure child is comfortable
- If outside hours, and not sent to the laboratory as a matter of urgency, use a preservative and store in specimen fridge
- Record the collection of specimen in the nursing documentation.

Safety issues
- In accordance with Universal Precautions, gloves should be worn for protection when involved in handling of body fluids
- When using a needle to aspirate sample, care and attention is required to avoid a needle stick injury
- If patient is possibly infected with a high-risk organism the specimen and request form should be labelled with biohazard tape. This procedure must be performed aseptically even if the sample requested need not be sterile. This is to avoid the introduction of infection into the catheter resulting in an ascending urine infection.

Adaptation for home care
- This procedure can be performed in the community following training given to parents.

Discussion point
- ❖ A urine sample may be requested for pregnancy test and/or drug toxicology. Consider the rights of the patient to full information and check if patient or parents, depending upon the age and condition of the child have given consent.

See *Appendix III*

Catheterisation of a female child

Definition: A method of emptying the bladder by using a urethral catheter

Purpose: The procedure enables the bladder to be emptied as a single or intermittent procedure.

Equipment required

- Sterile gloves
- Dressing pack
- 0.9% sodium chloride (warmed to 36–37°C)
- Lubricating jelly
- Urethral catheter
- Receiver dish
- Rubbish bag
- Toys suitable for age
- Specimen pot.

Additional equipment for indwelling catheter

- Syringe
- Needle
- Sterile water
- Spigot
- Drainage bag
- Adhesive plaster.

Psychological preparation and support

- Depending on the child's age, understanding and developmental level this procedure may possibly be viewed as intrusive and the child may be unco-operative
- Explanations of all procedures prior to undertaking the procedure are essential to help reduce the child's anxiety and maximise co-operation
- It is essential that a private area of ward/department be identified to undertake procedure.

Nursing interventions

- Explain procedure to the child and parents
- Lie infant/child in optimum position, normally supine with knees bent and flexed outwards
- Place protective undersheet under the buttocks
- Wash hands using Ayliffe Taylor method and put on sterile gloves
- Using cotton wool soaked in warmed saline, gently cleanse genital area in downward strokes. Gradually cleanse from outer to inner aspects of labia
- Position receiver close by
- On location of urethra, dip end of catheter tip into lubricating jelly and insert into urethra until urine escapes into receiver via catheter
- Gently palpate abdomen to remove any residual urine
- If this is a single procedure withdraw catheter slowly, observing for any further residual urine
- If catheter is to remain in situ, inflate catheter balloon with correct amount of water as indicated in product information
- Secure catheter
- Attach catheter bag or insert spigot
- Reposition child comfortably

- Clear away equipment and wash hands
- Take urine specimen if required.

Safety issues

- Enlist the help of family if the child is unco-operative
- Seek assistance if unable to locate urethra within two attempts
- Risk of shock due to large loss of urine: observe vital signs. Monitor urine output and inform medical staff.

Adaptation for home care

- Procedure can be undertaken in the home following training for child/parents/carers.

Further reading

Lowbury EJL, Ayliffe GA (eds) (1992) *Control of Hospital Infection.* 2nd edn. Chapman and Hall, London: Ch 7, 72–3

Birmingham Children's Hospital NHS Trust (1990) *Going Home.* Urodynamic Department booklet. 3rd edn. Birmingham Children's Hospital NHS Trust, Birmingham

See *Appendix III*

> *Nursing notes*

Chest drain, care of

Definition: Method of removing air/fluid from pleural cavity

Purpose: Safe maintenance of a closed underwater seal drainage system following insertion of a chest drain.

Equipment required

- Closed drainage system
- Two chest tube clamps
- Low pressure wall suction (as required)
- Fluid balance/chest drainage chart.

Psychological preparation and support

- Ensure child and family are aware of the reason for the insertion of the drain and the safety issues involved.

Nursing observations

Specific observations are:
- Chest drain site
- Condition of skin
- Signs of infection
- Signs of leakage
- Audible air leak.

Drainage:
- Type and amount of drainage
- Blood pressure (hypotension due to large or persistent drainage).

Nursing interventions

- Commence hourly recording of drainage (noting type and amount)
- Send specimens as required (M.C.+ S, Chyle)
- Ensure low pressure suction (3–5kpa) attached as per medical instructions — suction is usually indicated for most pleural drains
- Change drainage system aseptically when full or otherwise indicated. Drains can be reprimed daily if required
- Dress drain site as required.

Safety issues

- Ensure drainage system is adequately primed
- Use drain holders to ensure stability on the floor
- Always have two chest clamps with the patient at all times
- Keep drainage bottle below patient's chest level to prevent backflow of fluid
- If in doubt do not clamp the drain, unless the safety of the system cannot be guaranteed (as during transfer), and then only clamp as long as necessary
- If the patient has continuous air leak **do not** clamp the drain
- Milking (stripping) of the drain is only necessary to maintain patency; build-up of fibrin and clots can cause the drain to block (for advice on this technique ask experienced staff)

- Following insertion, length of drain at entry site should be noted in the nursing notes in case it becomes displaced
- Replacement fluid (usually 4.5% Human Albumin Solution) may be required following persistent losses or a sudden large fluid loss
- Inform medical staff if drain stops 'swinging' (usually means lung has reinflated) or if a continuous air leak starts
- Position tubing so it does not drag which can be painful and may dislodge the drain
- If drain becomes disconnected, clamp on patient side and contact medical staff; observe for bilateral chest movements and oxygen saturations.

Further reading

McMahon-Parkes K (1997) Management of pleural drains. *Nursing Times* 24 December **93**(52): 48–52

Erickson R (1989) Chest drainage part 1. *Nursing* May: 37–43

Erickson R (1998) Chest drainage part 2. *Nursing* June: 47–49

Walsh M (1989) Making sense of chest drainage. *Nursing Times* 14 June **85**(24): 40–41

Williams T (1992) To clamp or not to clamp. *Nursing Times* 29 April **88**(18):33

Campbell J (1993) Making sense of underwater sealed drainage. *Nursing Times* 3 March **89**(9): 34–36

Allan D (1985) Chest tube patients. *Nursing Times* 30 January: 24–25

See *Appendix III*

Nursing notes

Chest drain insertion

Definition: The insertion of drainage tube into the pleural cavity

Purpose: Chest drains are inserted for the purpose of removing air/fluid from the pleural or mediastinal space.

NB. This procedure should be carried out in theatre but on occasion it may be necessary to undertake it in a ward/department environment.

Equipment required

- Skin cleansing solution
- Local anaesthetic
- IV cutdown set
- Surgical blade (number 11 or 15)
- Suture (3° silk)
- Sterile drapes x two small
- Closed underwater seal drainage system
- 150mls sterile water for priming system
- Two chest drain clamps
- Specimen pot (microscopy, culture and sensitivity of pleural fluid)
- Oxygen.

Psychological preparation and support

- Explain the procedure at an appropriate level to the child's age and understanding
- Ensure that the child and carers understand that analgesia will be given regularly and as required
- Dependant on child's age, explain to child and carers the safety factors involved in the care of a chest drain (see care of a chest drain procedure).

Nursing observations

- Prior to procedure obtain baseline observations of temperature, pulse, respiration, blood pressure, oxygen saturation level, and patient's current weight
- If there is any fluid aspirated or drained record on patient's fluid balance chart, along with any fluid replacement that may be given
- During and initially after the procedure regular observation of the child's respiratory rate, oxygen saturation, pulse and blood pressure should be noted and recorded until the child's condition is stabilised
- Observation should be made of the drain site for any audible leak or excessive bleeding; a small gauze dressing is sufficient to cover around the wound site.

Nursing interventions

- Prior to the procedure ensure the child has patent IV access
- Intravenous sedation may be required, if so, it should be discussed with an anaesthetist
- Ensure adequate analgesia is prescribed and administered, even if sedation is used
- If the child is respiration is compromised, oxygen may be required during the procedure, if not it should be available for emergency use
- Commence oxygen and saturation recordings and non invasive blood pressure recordings during the procedure

- Fluid that is aspirated from the chest should be sent for MC & S and prophylactic antibiotics considered
- Note and record the amount and the type of fluid that is drained
- If hypotensive, colloid replacement (usually 4.5% H.A.S.) may be required
- Following insertion a chest x-ray should be taken
- According to the doctor's instructions low pressure suction (3–5kpa) may be applied to the drain
- Inform medical staff if the fluid stops 'swinging' or if it suddenly starts bubbling continuously or there is a change in the type or amount of drainage (heavily blood stained or milky fluid)
- A small gauze or occlusive dressing can be applied; change as necessary.

Safety issues

- Two chest drain clamps must be with the child at all times in case of accidental disconnection
- A note should be made of the length of the drain inserted, so if it slips the medical staff can be informed of the change
- Observation of the child following drain insertion is paramount; respiratory rate effort and pattern and bilateral air entry should be noted
- Drain must always be clamped on the drain side prior to disconnection
- Universal precautions should be observed
- When disconnecting the drain a clean technique should be used.

Further reading

McMahon-Parkes K (1997) Management of pleural drains. *Nursing Times* 24 December **93**(52): 48–52

Erickson R (1989) Chest drainage part 1. *Nursing* May: 37–43

Erickson R (1998) Chest drainage part 2. *Nursing* June: 47–49

Walsh M (1989) Making sense of chest drainage. *Nursing Times* 14 June **85**(24):40–41

Williams T (1992) To clamp or not to clamp. *Nursing Times* 29 April **88**(18): 33

Campbell J (1993) Making sense of underwater sealed drainage. *Nursing Times* 3 March **89**(9): 34–36

Allan D (1985) Chest tube patients. *Nursing Times* 30 January: 24–25

Discussion points

Clamping of drains:

❖ There is often confusion and controversy regarding the clamping of chest drains. These are some examples of when to clamp and when to avoid it. These are offered as guidelines only, as situations can change.

❖ The chest drains must always be kept below waist level to prevent back flow of fluid. If this is not possible, or the safety of the drains cannot be guaranteed, then clamps should be used. Chest drains do not routinely need to be clamped for transfer or movement of the patient.

❖ Two pairs of chest drain clamps must always be with the patient to use in case of disconnection or breakage of the bottle.

❖ Clamps should be applied to the patient side of the tubing, above the connection.

❖ Clamps should not be left on for long periods of time. As the child may be compromised by a collection of fluid or air.

❖ If a patient has a continuous air leak (drain is bubbling all the time) is must never be clamped, as a life-threatening pneumothorax can quickly develop.

Milking (stripping of drains)

❖ Mediastinal drains, which are inserted following cardiac or thoracic surgery, will need milking to maintain patency as long as they continue to drain.

❖ Pleural drains, as a rule, do not need milking unless they have been in situ for more than a few days as the formation of fibrin can cause the drain to block and milking may be required to maintain patency.

See *Appendix III*

Nursing notes

Colonic cone irrigation

Definition: A method of cleansing the colon via the rectum

Purposes: To achieve faecal continence where laxatives, suppositories or enemas have been unsuccessful. The frequency of the procedure will vary from child to child. To prevent soiling this procedure may be required daily, on alternate days or every third day.

Equipment required

- Toilet facilities
- Irrigation cone or bag
- Tubing
- Clamp
- Water
- Water holder
- Lubricating jelly
- Measuring jug
- Kitchen salt
- Teaspoon
- Lukewarm tap water
- Hook/drip stand
- Protective undersheet/blanket
- Disposable gloves.

Psychological preparation and support

- Explain procedure to child according to his/her level of understanding to promote trust and co-operation
- Consider the use of distraction therapy during initial aspects of procedure
- Privacy/screens
- Activities for younger child.

Nursing observations

- Record patient's weight to calculate fluid volume
- Observe skin surrounding anus
- Soiling — note when started and type of faecal matter
- On completion of procedure assist child with dressing and repositioning
- Wash irrigation set in detergent and hang up to dry
- Record outcome of procedure in nursing notes.

Nursing interventions

- If procedure is to take place as an inpatient contact stoma nurse specialist
- Explain procedure to child and family, incorporating their help and assistance as able
- Prepare irrigation fluid by mixing lukewarm tap water and salt in measuring jug
- Pour fluid into water holder, release clamp to allow fluid to prime line and expel air. Re-clamp
- Suspend water holder on hook/drip stand about one to two metres above child's hip level
- Lubricate tip of cone with jelly
- Assist child into correct position with child lying on left side with legs drawn up to chest

- Put on gloves
- Insert tip of cone into anus
- Release clamp and allow fluid to run in slowly. If leakage occurs gently insert cone tip further in until leakage stops
- Once all the fluid has run in, re-clamp tubing. Holding the cone in place, lift child onto the toilet
- Remove cone once child is seated on the toilet
- Child will need to sit for 30–45 minutes. During this time gentle massage of the abdomen will assist in ensuring all fluid is expelled.

> Fluid volume depends on weight of child:
> 20ml of water for every kilogram of body weight
> Add one teaspoon of salt for every 300ml of water measured

Safety issues

- Contact medical staff if child experiences the following:
  - rectal bleeding
  - retention of irrigation fluid.

> **Contraindication**
>
> ❖ Children with ano-rectal abnormalities are usually suitable candidates for this procedure. However, if child should have any of the following this procedure should not be undertaken:
>   - megacolon
>   - gut motility problems
>   - inflammatory bowel disease.

Adaptation for home care

- Procedure more likely to occur in home care situation.

Further reading

Myers C (1996) *Stoma Care Nursing — A Patient Centred Approach.* Arnolds, London: Ch 12
Oldham T, Colombian PM, Foglia RP (1997) *Surgery of Infants and Children: Scientific Principles and Practice.* Lippincott Raven, Philadelphia: Ch 83

See *Appendix III*

Enteral feeding: continuous feeding via a pump

Definition: A method of supplying nutrients via an enteral feeding pump

Purpose: To deliver feed safely.

Equipment required

- Pump
- Feed administration set
- Feed
- pH paper
- Alcohol wipes
- Trolley
- Syringe
  - 10ml or 50ml, depending on tube type
- Gallipot
- Disposable gloves
- Enteral feeding labels
- Sterile water
- Drip stand.

Psychological preparation and support

- Discuss the reasons for enteral feeding with parent/carer and child
- Assess age and developmental level of child/infant
- Give explanation of procedure to parent and child.

Best practice

- ❖ Development of oral feeding skills is essential for children receiving continuous feeds.
- ❖ For babies encourage mouth games at non-feeding times, eg. blowing kisses.
- ❖ For toddlers, sit child in a chair with feed-related toys to ensure feeding is a pleasurable experience.

Nursing observations

- If tube becomes blocked try flushing with warm water, lemonade or pineapple juice. (Pancreatic enzymes can be used if prescribed for unblocking tubes.) Liaise with dietetic colleague's regarding use of flushes
- Ensure child's weight is accurately recorded daily or as requested by dietetic colleagues. NB. All children should have an accurate height and weight recorded (head circumference if child under two) on admission
- If child develops diarrhoea please inform medical/dietetic staff
- Liquid part of stool should be sent immediately to clinical chemistry for reducing substances and microbiology, culture and sensitivity
- If child develops profuse vomiting, stop feed. Inform dietetic and medical staff. Observe child for signs of aspiration. Be prepared to resuscitate.

Nursing interventions

- Check child's identity band
- Check the prescribed feed/rate and expiry date against dietetic prescription.
  NB. Unused feed must be discarded after 24 hours
- Ensure a clean working surface is available
- Clean surfaces with alcohol wipes
- Clean enteral feeding pump
- Check alarms are functioning
- Clean top of the feed container with alcohol impregnated wipes
- If a can opener is to be used wash and clean with alcohol impregnated wipes
- Wash hands
- Put on disposable gloves
- In the use of sterile feeds fill reservoir with total volume to be given. Ensure you do not contaminate the inside of the reservoir.
  NB. Modular feeds — if there are additives in the feed please refill reservoir every four hours
- Prime the feeding line
- Insert feed line into pump ensuring it is well secured
- Check position of tube in place
- Nasogastric
  - aspirate tube and test acidity using pH paper 0–6 pH. NB. Some feeds in use are acidic, ensure fluid is taken from the stomach
- Gastrostomy
  - leave the tube on free drainage, test acidity as above 0–6 pH
- Jejunostomy
  - use pH paper to assess alkalinity < 6.0
- If there are problems with placement of tube — reposition
- To ensure oral skills develop, if possible let the child have something in their mouth to taste/suck while they are tube fed
- Flush feeding tube with minimal amount of sterile water to ensure patency.

Further reading

Anderton A, Nivgough CE (1991) Problems with the re-use of enteral feeding systems. A study of the effectiveness of a range of cleaning and disinfection procedures. *Journal of Human Nutrition and Dietetics* **4**: 25–32

Baker SB, Baker RD, Davis A (1994) *Paediatric Enteral Nutrition* . Chapman and Hall, London

Holden CE, MacDonald A, Ward M, Ford K *et al* (1997) Psychological preparation for nasogastric feeding in children. *British Journal of Nursing* **6**(7): 376–85

Holden C, Sexton E, Paul L (1997) Enteral nutrition for children. *Nursing Standard* **11**(32): 49–54

Holden C, MacDonald A (1997) Nutritional Support at home: Emotional support and composition of feeds. *Current Paediatric* **7**:18–22

Metheny N, Williams P, Wiersema L, Wherle MS *et al* (1989) Effectiveness of pH measurements on predicting feeding tube placement. *Nursing Research* **38**: 280–85

Metheny N, Reed L, Wiersema L, McSweaney M *et al* (1993) Effectiveness in predicting feeding tube placement: An update. *Nursing Research* **42**(6): 324–31

Metheny N, Reed L, Clarke J, Worseck M (1993) How to aspirate fluid from small bore feeding tubes. *American Journal of Nursing* **93**: 86–8

Patchell CJ, Anderton A, MacDonald A, George RH, Booth IW (1994) Bacterial contamination of enteral feeds. *Archives of Diseases in Childhood* **70**: 327–30

Sexton E, Paul L, Holden CE (1997) Pictorial teaching aid for parents. *Paediatric Nursing* **8**(5): 24–6

See *Appendix III*

Nursing notes

Eye care

Definition: The process of cleansing the outer eye

Purpose: To prevent eye infections and provide patient comfort.

Equipment required

- Disposable gloves
- Sodium chloride sachets 0.9%
- Sterile gauze swab
- Eye medication, if prescribed
- Dressing pack and two gallipots
- Trolley
- Geliperm
- Sterile blade.

Psychological preparation and support

- Assess age and developmental level of child
- Assess parents/carers understanding of relevance of eye care and if they wish to participate
- Explain procedure.

Nursing observations

- Prior to cleansing eye assess condition of eye, surrounding skin and eyelashes.

Nursing interventions

- Ensure adequate, but not excessive bright light for procedure
- Assist child in finding comfortable position
- Clean trolley surface
- Wash hands and open pack. Arrange equipment to be used
- Wash hands using Ayliffe Taylor method and place on gloves
- Fold gauze swab and soak in sodium solution. Remove excess moisture from swab
- Begin with the 'clean' eye and wipe the eyelid from the inner canthus to the outer canthus. Discard swab
- Repeat cleansing procedure as necessary for each eye
- Instil prescribed eye drops/ointment
- Remove gloves and discard equipment and wash hands
- Assist child with repositioning.

Unconscious child

- Assess the condition of the eye, eyelashes and lids and surrounding skin
- Cleanse eyes as per procedure, beginning with cleanest eye first
- If crusting persists lay damp swab across eyelid for a few seconds
- Once eyelid and eyelashes are clean, raise upper eyelid and examine eye
- Assess condition of conjunctiva and cornea and need for artificial protection
- For dry or swollen corneas instil eye ointment along the lower eyelid from inner to outer canthus
- For incomplete closure, cut two squares of Geliperm large enough to cover upper and lower eyelid.

Safety issues

- Each tube/bottle of ointment/drops should be individually labelled left and right eye and dated on opening
- Some infections can cause permanent damage, eg. Pseudomonas Aeruginosa. If an infection is suspected contact medical staff.

Potential problems

- Purulent discharge: Inform medical staff
- Take swab from each eye and send for microbiology, culture and sensitivity
- Administer topical antibiotics as prescribed
- Continue with eye care as frequently as required to maintain patient comfort.

Adaptation for home care

- The principles of the procedure can be undertaken in the home.

Further reading

Farrell M, Wray F (1993) Eye care for ventilated patients. *Intensive and Critical Care Nursing* (9): 137–41

Lloyd F (1990) Making sense of eye care for ventilated or unconscious patients. *Nursing Times* **86**(1): 36–7

Sutton T (1993) Research in practice: eye care. *Paediatric Nursing* **5**(3): 23

See *Appendix III*

Nursing notes

Eye swab

Definition: The collection of a sample of exudate from the eye for the purpose of laboratory examination

Purpose: To obtain a sample for laboratory study to determine the presence and specific type of micro-organism.

Equipment required

- 0.9% sodium chloride
- Dry sterile specimen swab
- To moisten swab, if required
- Disposable gloves
- Culture medium, if required, eg. swab is not sent to laboratory immediately
- Request form
- Items required for eye cleansing.

Psychological preparation and support

- Assess child's age and understanding when explaining and preparing for procedure
- Involve the parents/carer
- The procedure may be performed with child sitting in a chair or bed, on carer's lap, or lain down.

Nursing observations

- Observe the eyes for redness, swelling and obvious exudate
- Note if specimen from one eye only is required, or both
- This procedure should be performed prior to eye care being given.

Nursing intervention

- Explain procedure to child and carer(s)
- Check child's identity against request form
- Prepare equipment
- Label swab container with child's name, registration number and ward
- Position child comfortably, so that head can be supported
- Wash hands using Ayliffe Taylor method
- Put on gloves
- Moisten tip of swab with sterile saline
- Gently apply swab to external eye area using one 'stroke', collecting a sample of any exudate or pus present
- Carefully replace the swab in the designated container and seal
- Obtain swab from other eye if required
- Proceed to perform eye care/cleansing
- Dispose of gloves and wash hands
- Assist child in maintaining comfortable position
- Note that the time of sample collection is written on the request form and specimen, indicating whether taken from left or right eye
- Secure together and send to laboratory
- Record collection of sample in nursing documentation

- If sample is collected outside laboratory hours, place in a culture medium and store in specimen fridge.

Safety issues

- Care is needed when collecting sample to avoid injury to the eye
- If eye is not visibly moist, the swab must be pre-moistened to avoid leaving a residue of micro-fibre in the eye area
- In accordance with Universal Precautions gloves are worn
- If patient is possibly infected with a high-risk organism, specimen and request form should be labelled with biohazard tape.

Adaptation for home care

- This procedure may be carried out in the home.

Further reading

Lloyd F (1990) Making sense of eye care for ventilated or unconscious patients. *Nursing Times* **86**(1): 36–7

Sutton T (1993) Research in practice: eye care. *Paediatric Nursing* **5**(3): 23

See *Appendix III*

> *Nursing notes*

Fresh frozen plasma (FFP), collection and administration

Definition: Citrated plasma separated from whole blood, all coagulation factors preserved (usually stored frozen for up to twelve months)

Purpose: Fresh frozen plasma is used to treat bleeding episodes or to prepare patients for surgery in certain defined situations.

Equipment required
- Identification form
- Prescription chart
- IV administration set
- IV pump
- Water bath/warmer.

Psychological preparation and support
- Inform child and carers reason for infusion appropriate to age and development
- Consider whether religious observances may impact on the initiation of this treatment.

Nursing observations
- Record infusion of plasma on a fluid balance chart and in nursing notes
- Observe infusion site for patency throughout administration
- Record observations of blood pressure, temperature, pulse and respiration as per blood transfusion procedure
- Ensure batch number of blood products administered are documented in medical/nursing notes.

Nursing interventions
- Take completed identification form to Blood Bank (ensure access can be gained out of hours, ie. know the door code or porter)
- Complete FFP registration folder in Blood Bank (including legible signature)
- File identification form at collection point
- On return to the ward FFP should be thawed immediately in a 37°C water bath and used within two hours of thawing
- Observing Universal Precautions and Trust policy, relating to Intravenous Drug Administration, commence infusion as prescribed
- If unused, return FFP to Blood Bank but do not re-freeze. Inform haematologist.

Safety issues
- Must be fully thawed
- Must be used within two hours
- Ensure universal procedures are followed
- Disposal of blood products.

Adaptation for home care
- Not applicable.

See *Appendix III*

Gastrostomy button device (skin level device)

Definition: The insertion of a skin level device directly into the stomach

Purpose: To safely insert the correct sized device into the stomach for feeding.
NB. An established tract must be formed prior to gastrostomy button insertion.

Equipment required

- Button stoma measuring device
- Dressing pack
- 0.9% sodium chloride solution
- Soluble lubricant
- Disposable gloves
- 10mls syringe
- Litmus paper
- Sterile water
- Analgesia as required.

Psychological preparation and support

- Explain to the child and family the need for the insertion of the gastrostomy button to enhance their understanding and co-operation
- Assess child's and family's understanding of procedure
- Assess age and developmental level of the infant/child to facilitate correct psychological preparation prior to insertion of the gastrostomy button device.

Nursing observations

- Clean stoma site with warm saline solution and dry thoroughly to prevent infection
- Inspect the stoma site routinely for any irregularities (ie. redness, swelling or discomfort). Twice a day lift the edges of button device and gently clean around the stoma site. Dry thoroughly
- Rotate button 360 degrees daily to prevent tissue adherence to the button
- Leakage of feed around button: check for correct balloon inflation
- To prevent gastrostomy button blockage, use liquid medicines if at all possible
- Flush button device before and after giving medicines with sterile water.

Check placement and patency prior to administration of drugs or feed

- Use extension set provided and connect up to button. Aspirate for gastric contents using blue litmus paper to turn pink. Alternatively pH paper to be used and scored on a scale of one to six. Check for ease of flushing.
- **When patency is assured, open the feeding port of extension set to allow air to escape. This ensures stomach is free of wind and air prior to feeding.**

Feeding administration

- Open the plug on the button to reveal the anti-reflux valve, connect feeding system up using extension set provided, as per Trust policy. (Bolus feeding/Continuous feeding protocols in the *Procedure Manual*.)

Nursing interventions

- Give analgesia as prescribed
- Wash hands thoroughly prior to handling device. Put on gloves
- Remove stoma-measuring device from package
- Moisten the tip of the measuring device with soluble lubricant or water
- Deflate balloon by attaching syringe to sidearm and withdraw water
- Gently remove the existing gastrostomy tube/button device and discard
- Support the child's abdomen
- Insert the device through the stoma to the stomach. **Do not use force**, approximately 2.5–3.7 cm (1–1.5 inches). Inflate the balloon with 5mls of water
- Gently pull on the stoma-measuring device until you can feel resistance against the stomach wall
- Position the child in a supine stoma position and slide the plastic disk down to the stoma
- Read the marking at the top of the disc then add 1–2mm to the actual stoma length
- Slide the disk out away from the stoma and raise the baby/child to an upright position
- Slide the disk down to the stoma
- Read the marking at the top of the disk
- Take an average of the two readings. This is the desired length
- Record the measurement on shaft length
- Deflate the balloon and remove the device

Placement of skin level device

- Using a level tip syringe inflate the balloon with 5mls of sterile water. If the balloon is not symmetrical, gently manipulate it by rolling the balloon between your fingers or palms of hands until it frees itself. This is done to ensure button device is working properly
- Deflate the balloon
- Lubricate the tip of the tube with water-soluble lubricant and gently guide the tube through the stoma and into the stomach
- Inflate the balloon with 3–5mls of sterile water to ensure the balloon is held in position against the stomach wall
- Gently lift the edge of the button device and check for signs of gastric leakage
- If leakage is observed increase the balloon volume by 2mls. (**Do not** exceed 5ml volume in the balloon.)

Safety issues

- Unable to place device
- Do not force — ensure child's abdomen is relaxed. Use smaller sized tube
- Inform senior nursing staff or surgical medical team so that appropriate size tube can be inserted
- Please ensure a tube or button is inserted immediately to prevent stoma from closing
- Frequency of changing button device. Please refer to manufacturer instructions (approximately five to six months).

Adaptation for home care

- The procedure remains the same except boiled water, which has been allowed to cool, can be used at home for flushing purposes
- The procedure is conducted as above by trained nursing staff or parents who have been assessed by community or hospital staff.

Further reading

Holden C, Babb Y, Sexton E (2000) *Guidelines for the Care of the Mic-Key Skin Level Gastrostomy Kit.* Birmingham Children's Hospital NHS Trust, Vygon UK Ltd, Gloucester

Haas-Beckett B, Heymon MB (1993) Comparison of two skin-level gastrostomy feeding tubes for infants and children. *Paediatric Nursing* **19**(9): 351–4, 424

Holden CE , Sexton E, Caney D, Fitzpatrick D (1997) *Gastrostomy Reference Guide.* Nutritional Care Department, Birmingham Children's Hospital NHS Trust, Birmingham

Holden C, Fitzpatrick G, Paul L, Sexton E *et al* (1997). *Gastrostomy Care – Parents*. Nutritional Care Department, Birmingham Children's Hospital NHS Trust, Birmingham

Malki TA, Langer JC, Thompson V, McQueen M *et al* (1991) A prospective evaluation of the button gastrostomy in children. *Canadian Journal of Surgery* **34**: 247–50

Nutritional Care Department (1997) Mic-Key factsheet. Birmingham Children's Hospital NHS Trust, Birmingham

Taylor S, Goodinson-McLaren S (1992) Nasoenteral and enterostomy feeding. In: *Nutritional Support: A team approach.* Wolfe Publishing Ltd, London

See *Appendix III*

Nursing notes

Gastrostomy tube change

Definition: The insertion of a gastrostomy tube directly into the stomach

Purpose: To safely insert a gastrostomy tube through an established tract into the stomach.

Equipment required

- Gastrostomy tube
- 0.9% sodium chloride sachet/sterile water
- Dressing pack
- 10ml syringe x two
- Water soluble lubricant
- Disposable gloves
- Litmus paper/pH paper
- Connector and cap if required.

Psychological preparation and support

- Assess age and developmental level of the infant/child in order to facilitate correct psychological preparation prior to inserting the gastrostomy button device
- Discuss support for child with play therapy department
- Explain to the child and family the need for the insertion of the gastrostomy tube to enhance their understanding and co-operation
- Assess child's and family's understanding of procedure.

Nursing observations

- Inspect (the stoma) enterostomy site daily and clean with warm saline solution
- If the skin around stoma is inflamed or shows leakage, discharge or granulation tissue, swab site and send to microbiology. Inform medical staff. Refer to Trust Policy 1997 Gastrostomy site problems
- Leakage of feed around gastrostomy tube
  - Check water in balloon with 10ml syringe, if less then 3mls of water instil sterile water to maximum of five minutes into valve. Recheck volume
- Tube migrating into small bowel
  - Pull tube back gently until resistance is felt. Tape tube securely to abdomen to prevent tube slipping back
- Tube falls out
  - This procedure can be potentially uncomfortable and distressing. It is therefore important to observe the child's general well-being and level of anxiety. Give support and reassurance as well as explaining each step of the procedure. Replace tube if you have been shown how to do this. Contact senior nursing staff/medical staff/nutritional care sisters immediately since the stoma closes off within a few hours
- If unable to insert the same size tube. Please revert to using a smaller tube for 24 hours. Re-insert correct size the next day or as able
- Leakage around the site may be a result of the secure lock ring not being properly adjusted, if in use. The balloon must be against the stomach wall
- The tube and any lock ring should be cleaned daily with warm saline solution. Failure to do so results in build up of debris, risking contamination and oily deposits
- The tube should be flushed with sterile water before and after medications or feeds.

Nursing interventions

- Ensure feed is switched off/discontinued prior to tube change
- Give analgesia/sedation as prescribed. Topical analgesia preparations can also be used
- Wash hands
- Assemble all equipment required for changing the tube, open dressing pack
- Put on gloves
- Remove the new tube from the plastic sleeve
- Check balloon patency of new tube by attaching a syringe filled with saline onto the sidearm of the catheter. Fill with 3–5mls sterile water or saline. If necessary roll the catheter-inflated balloon gently between the thumb and the index finger until it inflates symmetrically, then deflate
- Attach 10ml syringe to sidearm of established tube and gently withdraw all water. The balloon will deflate and the tube is then ready to come out
- Position the thumb and forefinger 5cm (2 inches) apart either side of the gastrostomy to stabilise the exit site
- Gently pull the tube out
- Clean the stoma site with warm solution saline
- Moisten the end of the tube with a water soluble lubricant, do not use petroleum jelly. Gently guide the catheter through the stoma about 2.5–3.7 cm (1–1.5 inches infants and children) or until the entire balloon has passed through the tract
- A balloon catheter should be gently pulled until slight tension is felt as the balloon comes against the stomach wall. The length of the tube external to the stoma should be noted and marked. Tubes without retention discs must be taped firmly to prevent movement of the tube down into the duodenum. If in use slide retention discs/secure locks within 1–2mm of skin surface
- Insert connector and cap into the end of tube (if required)
- Attach 10ml syringe and draw back stomach juice and test on blue litmus paper for pink reaction, pH paper to be used if child is receiving antacids. Acidic 1–6 pH
- Flush gastrostomy tubes with 3–5mls sterile cooled water and attach cap.

Safety issues

- Difficulty in flushing may be an indication that the tube is blocked or incorrectly positioned. Always test acidity with litmus to ensure correct placement. Use pH paper
- If the child develops pain, discomfort or diarrhoea,
  - It may be as a result of the tube being delivered directly into the duodenum. Ensure balloon is against the stomach wall. Check correct volume of water has been used to inflate tube. Over inflation can lead to migration into intestine and lead to obstruction. Always secure tube at skin surface (if retention disc not available)
- It is only applicable to remove and replace gastrostomy tubes with balloon type inflation. PEG tubes (percutaneous endoscopic gastrostomy tubes) which have a silicone limiting disc/buffer to prevent extubation will be replaced by surgeons in theatre
- Frequency of changing tubes will be dependent upon tube type (usually 3–4 monthly). Refer to manufacturer's instructions.

Adaptation for home care

- Procedure remains the same except boiled water, which has been allowed to cool, can be used at home for flushing purposes. Qualified nursing staff must teach parents prior to discharge.

Further reading

Holden C, Fitzpatrick G, Paul L, Sexton E *et al* (1997) *Gastrostomy Care:A Parents Guide.* Nutritional Care Department, Birmingham Children's Hospital NHS Trust, Birmingham

Rombeau JL, Caldwell MD, Forlaw L, Guenter PA (1989) *Atlas of Nutritional Support Techniques.* Little Brown Co, Boston

Taylor S, Goodinson-McLaren S (1992) Nasoenteral and enterostomy feeding In: *Nutritional Support: A Team Approach.* Wolfe Publishing Ltd, London

See *Appendix III*

Nursing notes

Isolation of childhood infectious diseases

Infection	Precautions	Duration of isolation
Bronchiolitis	Respiratory	For the duration of the clinical illness
Chickenpox, shingles	Respiratory (Chickenpox only) Excretion/Secretion (vesicle fluid)	Until vesicles have all crusted
Gartro-enteritis, rotavirus	Enteric Respiratory	Until virological tests show rotavirus no longer present
Gastro-enteritis, other viruses or unknown aetiology	Enteric Respiratory	Until asymptomatic for 48 hours
Group A streptococcus (Streptococcus pyogenes)	Skin/Wound Respiratory	Until after 48 hours appropriate antibiotic treatment
Haemolytic uraemic syndrome	Enteric	Source isolation until no diarrhoea for 48 hours. Continue enteric precautions until advised by ICT
Haemophilus influenzae type b (Hib) disease	Respiratory	Until after 48 hours appropriate antibiotic treatment
Hand, foot and mouth disease	Respiratory Excretion/Secretion (vesicle fluid)	For the duration of the clinical illness
Hepatitis A	Enteric	Until one week after onset of jaundice
Influenza	Respiratory	For the duration of the clinical illness
Measles	Respiratory	Until five days after onset of the rash
Meningococcal disease	Respiratory	Until after 48 hours appropriate antibiotic treatment
Mumps	Respiratory	Until nine days after the onset of swelling
Pertusis	Respiratory	Until 21 days after the onset of paroxysmal cough or until seven days erythromycin therapy
Rubella	Respiratory	Until seven days after onset of the rash
Scabies	Skin/Wound	Following 24 hours following treatment
Tuberculosis	Respiratory	Until advised by ICT
Typhoid, paratyphoid fever	Enteric Excretion/Secretion (urine)	For the duration of hospital admission

Isolation of childhood infectious diseases

Injections (SC/IM)

Definition: A method of administrating medication using a hypodermic needle via the subcutaneous or intramuscular route

Purpose: To administer medication when no other method of administration is appropriate.

Equipment required

- Prescription chart
- Drug to be administered
- Tray
- Syringe/insulin, 0.5ml microfine syringe
- 1–2.5mls
- Needles x 2 23g/25g (one larger needle for ease of drawing up drug)
- Alcohol swab — for single use
- Cotton wool
- Plaster.

Psychological preparation and support

- Explain procedures according to developmental level of the child, allowing the child to express their fears, and ask any questions
- Consider the use of topical anaesthetic
- As necessary, involve play to explain procedure, ie. dolls
- Perform procedure as soon as possible after explanation, so as not to prolong anxiety
- Use appropriate encouragement and praise following procedure.

Nursing observations

- Identify injection site
- Major nerves and blood vessels must be avoided
- Larger amount of fluid, larger muscle needed
- Regular use of one site can cause fibrosis of the muscle
- Take care not to strike bone as needle inserted
- If blood is aspirated withdraw needle and repeat procedure
- Select the correct needle to the volume of fluid being administered and the smaller the needle, the more painful the administration.

Nursing interventions

- Prepare drug(s) in selected syringes and needle
- Wash hands using Ayliffe Taylor method
- Explain procedure to child, parents
- Position child in a comfortable, relaxed position, in a safe and secure way held by nurse or parent
- Identify area for injection
- Ensure area is clean and not restricted
- Wipe skin with alcohol swab. Allow to dry

- Administer drug as follows:

Subcutaneous
- pinch a fold of skin
- insert needle at 45° angle
- administer drug
- release pinch
- withdraw needle
- wipe clean with cotton wool
- apply pressure if leaking

Intramuscular
- stretch skin
- insert needle at a 90° angle
- leave a third of the needle shaft exposed
- withdraw plunger if no blood appears
- administer drug
- withdraw needle
- for intramuscular injection massage site to distribute drug
- cover with plaster if appropriate
- praise child appropriately and comfort
- record administration, note site administered

Safety issues

- Observe for reaction to the drug, ie. anaphylactic shock
- Be aware of potential needle-stick injuries and dispose of needles appropriately.

Adaptation for home care

- A nurse, parent, or child could perform the same procedure.

Discussion point

❖ Paediatric practice does not advocate use of injections except where this is the most effective and appropriate method of administration

---

Further reading

Brunner LS, Suddarth DS, Weller BF (1986) *The Lippincott Manual of Paediatric Nursing.* 2nd edn. Harper Row Ltd, London

Pritchard AP, Mallett J (1992) *The Royal Marsdon Hospital Manual of Clinical Nursing Procedures.* 3rd edn. The Royal Marsdon Hospital, London

Wellor BF (1990) *Ballière's Nurses Dictionary.* Ballière Tindall, London

Wong WL (1993) *Essentials of Paediatric Nursing.* 4th edn. Mosby, St Louis

See *Appendix III*

Last offices for a child/young person

Definition: The immediate care given to a child/young person following confirmation of death by medical staff

Purpose: To care for the body in a sensitive manner prior to transfer to mortuary.

Equipment required

- Washbowl
- Soap and water
- Towels
- Apron
- Nappy (if appropriate)
- Gloves
- Two name band's
- Gown or preferred clothing
- Comb/brush
- Clean linen
- Cotton wool
- Notice of death documentation
- Personal property documentation
- Body bag (if required).

Psychological preparation and support

- Family viewing: contact Bereavement Officer and porters to arrange
- Accompany carers where necessary
- Out of hours viewing: contact Duty Manager and accompany family to mortuary
- Most Trusts have produced a bereavement package which is available in all clinical areas
- Ensure family, friends and carers are as involved as possible.

Nursing intervention

- Ensure child has two name bands and that they are attached
- Consult the family on whether any particular religious observances should be performed
- Cleanse, dry and dress child in preferred clothing
- Remove any cannulas, catheters or drains which may be in situ
- Change bed linen and straighten body into supine position
- Close eyes (cover temporarily with wet cotton wool if eyes will not stay closed)
- If parents have been unable to participate, place toy/flower with child and remain close by while parents view body
- According to family wishes, other personal items of the child may be included at the viewing or transferred with the child to the mortuary, eg. football shirt, toys or gift from sibling
- After viewing, prepare child for transfer to mortuary by wrapping securely in white sheet leaving child's wristband easily accessible
- Enclose body in a transparent body bag if there is a risk of infection
- Liaise with the Bereavement Officer.

Transfer to mortuary

- Depending on the age and size of the child they maybe carried in parent's arms or lain in a pram or porter's trolley for transfer to mortuary.

Supply of body bags
- All children who have a high-risk infectious condition (HIV, Hepatitis) prior to death should be enclosed in a body bag
- Clear identification of the child's identity should be attached to the outside of the bag
- Body bags are available in a variety of sizes and may be ordered through a non-stock requisition. It would be preferable if a translucent type were ordered to facilitate identification of child.

Adaptation for home care
- This procedure is not recommended for home care although it is recognised that carers in the home will undertake some aspects of last offices.

Further reading

Lothian Community Relations Council, Edinburgh. Religions and Cultures (1994) *A Guide to Patients' Beliefs and Customs of Health Service Staff*, revised edition

Rodgers J (1987) Helping student nurses cope with patient deaths. *Nursing Times* **83**(40): 54

Walker C (1982) Attitudes to death and bereavement among cultural minority groups. *Nursing Times* December **78**(50): 2106–9

Walker C (1986) Easing the pain of bereaved parents. *Nursing* April: 49–50

Ahrens W, Hart R, Maruyama N (1997) Paediatric Death: managing the aftermath in the emergency department. *The Journal of Emergency Medicine* **15**(5): 601–3

See *Appendix III*

Nursing notes

Lumbar puncture

Definition: Insertion of a needle into the lumbar subarachnoid space

Purpose: To obtain cerebrospinal fluid for diagnostic or therapeutic purposes, or
to administer medication.

Equipment required

- Dressing trolley
- Spinal needles
- Dressing pack/lumbar puncture pack
- Sterile gloves
- Specimen bottles x three
  - microscopy
  - culture and sensitivity
  - glucose content
- Antiseptic cleansing solution
- 2ml syringes
- Local anaesthetic, eg. 1% lignocaine, if required, plus needle and syringe
- Waterproof plaster.

Psychological preparation and support

- Lumbar puncture is a painful procedure. If able, consider opportunities to provide information and preparation for child and family prior to procedure
- Establish whether parents wish to be present or not
- Talk to and reassure child throughout procedure to encourage comfort and promote safety, explaining each step of the procedure
- Following this procedure reposition child to more usual position offering reassurance and praise to child.

Nursing observations

- Note any increased/decreased respiratory effect, ie. level of chest expansion, oxygen saturation rate, pulse and respiratory rate
- Implementing procedure with a very distressed child may be inadvisable as procedure could lead to further trauma. Child may require sedation first
- Following lumbar puncture observe for signs of infection
- Due to spinal cord's association with brain function, monitor neurological status
- Administer analgesia as prescribed, monitoring its effectiveness
- Observe wound dressing for signs of leakage
- Consider whether pre-medication/sedation prior to undertaking procedure is appropriate
- Position child in lateral position at edge of bed, with knees drawn upwards and head forward, with chin resting on chest as if curling into a ball shape, with lumbar region exposed
- Ensure this position is maintained securely during procedure to enable maximum access to intervertebral spaces and to prevent sudden movement of infant/child
- Doctor will cleanse skin and apply local anaesthetic if necessary
- Spinal needle is inserted and once in place drips of CSF can be seen at needle tip
- Collect between 5–10 drops for each specimen bottle. Label/number each bottle consecutively 1,2,3
- Following removal of needle, apply firm pressure to wound and apply adhesive dressing.

Possible complications

- Herniation of brain stem
- Infection
- Leakage of CSF
- Respiratory distress
- Nerve damage.

Discussion point

❖ Some children have experienced post lumbar puncture headache, which is thought to relate to CSF being removed. In the past bed rest was commonly advocated but appears to have had little effect and is no longer routinely suggested.

Adaption for home care

- This procedure is not appropriate to be undertaken at home.

Further reading

Tobias JD (1996) Post dural puncture headache in children. *Headache Quarterly Current Treatment and Research* **7**(4): 306–11

Bassett C (1997) Medical Investigations 1: Lumbar Puncture. *British Journal of Nursing* **6**(7): 405–6

Whaley LF, Wang DL (1993) *Essentials of Paediatric Nursing.* Mosby, St Louis

Allan D (1989) Making sense of lumbar puncture. *Nursing Times* **85**(49): 39–41

See *Appendix III*

Nursing notes

Management of power sourced medical equipment

Definition: A medical device is any health care product requiring an energy source, eg. electricity/charged battery, which is used for a patient/client in the diagnosis, treatment, prevention or alleviation of illness or injury.

Purpose: To ensure items of equipment are correctly operated and that equipment is maintained.

Equipment required

- Items of equipment
- Electrical leads/charged batteries as required.

Nursing interventions

- Ensure equipment is clean and fit for use. Check for evidence of wear and tear. Do not use if it appears to be unfit for purpose
- Where able to install equipment at bedside prior to use, ensure it is correctly connected to electrical mains or new battery
- Check alarm systems, if present, are functioning. Calibrate equipment at each change of shift or as specified by the manufacturer
- As new items of equipment are introduced into a child's care, a record should be entered into the nursing notes. This record should include the product type, product name and serial number
- Where the rate or item of equipment has been altered or replaced, these changes should be documented in the nursing record.

Safety issues

- On receipt of new equipment it should go to a medical engineers department for:
  - entry into asset register
  - labelling
  - safety test prior to use
- Prior to introducing a new item of equipment to clinical area, relevant training should be arranged and implemented for staff required to operate equipment
- Should equipment require maintenance, the following actions actions should be taken:
  - cleanse equipment in line with decontamination procedure in the control of the infection policy
  - label equipment as not suitable for current use, specify fault if known
  - complete a request for maintenance by telephoning the medical engineer department and give details of fault and equipment identification number.

Potential problems

Alarm system generates a false alarm or does not alarm when it may have been expected to

- Action
  - withdraw equipment from use immediately
  - complete untoward incident form
  - contact Health and Safety Officer
  - label equipment as faulty, indicating where possible nature of the fault
  - document in nursing records.

Adaptation for home care

- The procedure may be undertaken in the community. In addition, families should be given information about who to contact should their equipment become faulty or require maintenance and on how to obtain replacements
- Equipment being used at home should register with the MEB in case of loss of power supply.

See *Appendix III*

Nursing notes

Mid-stream urine specimen collection

Definition: The collection of a urine sample for the purpose of investigation

Purpose: To obtain an uncontaminated sample of urine. As little as 2ml of urine may be sufficient for culture, 0.5ml for urine electrolytes. For more extensive clinical chemistry tests 10ml is required.

Equipment required

- Toilet/bathroom facilities
- Soap, water and towel
- Sterile container to initially collect the sample of urine
- Universal specimen pot — this may need to contain preservative, if the sample is to be cultured but not sent to the laboratory immediately
- Request form
- Non-sterile gloves.

Psychological preparation and support

- This method of urine collection is suitable for a continent child, with full assistance for pre-school and young children, and minimal supervision for older children/adolescents able to comply
- Privacy is paramount, particularly for the older child. Those requiring assistance or supervision are likely to prefer the input of a parent or primary carer.

Nursing observations

- Check that the sample is collected at the requested time (an early morning sample may be required)
- Assess the genital area during the cleansing process, noting any soreness, particularly signs of candida
- Note if the child experiences any pain or discomfort when voiding urine
- Observe the urine for any cloudiness or colour irregularity. Colour changes may be due to concentrated urine, or presence of blood or bilirubin. Cloudy urine may be due to urine infection or presence of protein
- Without contaminating a sterile sample, ward test urine if indicated or if it has not been done previously.

Nursing interventions

- Explain procedure to child, involving parents if present
- Check identity of child against the request form
- Label universal pot with child's details
- Ensure privacy
- Wash hands and apply gloves
- Wearing gloves, cleanse and dry the genital area, the child/adolescent may have a bath to do this
- Take child to the toilet or potty
- Ideally, the patient, parent or nurse should allow the initial urine flow to pass into the toilet, and collect the 'mid-stream' into the sterile collecting receptacle, wearing gloves to do so
- For a small child, unable to control flow, it is acceptable to place the sterile container into the potty or into a bowl in the toilet, then get child to sit down and pass urine

- With the nurse still wearing gloves, decant the urine into the laboratory specimen pot
- Assist/supervise child with dressing and hand washing, as appropriate
- Send to laboratory with request form, ensuring that the details are complete, including the date and time of urine sample, and the method of collection used (mid-stream) urine. If outside laboratory hours, and not requested as an urgent sample, use a pot containing preservative and store in specimen fridge
- Record the collection of specimen in the nursing documentation.

Safety issues

- Gloves should be worn for protection when involved in intimate cleansing or handling of body fluids
- If patient is possibly infected with a high-risk organism, specimen and request form should be labelled with biohazard tape.

Adaptation for home care

- Procedure for the collection of urine remains the same.

Discussion points

❖ Not all urine samples need to be collected sterile. If sample is not for microscopy, culture and sensitivity, then it may be satisfactory to collect urine from a clean (rather than sterile) receptacle.

❖ A urine sample (non-sterile) may be requested for pregnancy test and/or drug toxicity. Consider the rights of the patient to full information and check if consent has been given by the patient or parents.

See *Appendix III*

Nursing notes

Nasal swab

Definition: The collection of a sample of nasal secretions for the purpose of laboratory examination

Purpose: To obtain a sample for laboratory study to determine the presence and specific type of micro-organism.

Equipment required

- Dry sterile specimen swab
- Sterile saline to moisten swab
- Non-sterile gloves
- Culture medium, for use if swab is not sent to laboratory immediately
- Request form.

Psychological preparation and support

- Assess child's age and understanding when explaining and preparing for procedure
- Involve the parents if available
- Procedure may be done with child sat upright in chair or bed, sat on carer's lap, or lay in bed.

Nursing observations

- Observe the nasal area for signs of soreness
- Note if child's nose is particularly 'runny' and/or colour and consistency of secretions.

Nursing interventions

- Explain procedure to child and parents/carers
- Check child's identity against request
- Prepare equipment
- Label swab container with child's name, registration number and ward
- Position child as comfortably as possible with head tipped back
- Wash hands using Ayliffe Taylor method
- Put on gloves
- Moisten swab with sterile saline. This may not be necessary if there are obvious nasal secretions
- Insert the tip of the swab into the nasal cavity and gently rotate
- Withdraw the swab, taking care to avoid touching the skin
- Carefully replace the swab in the designated container and seal
- Dispose of gloves and wash hands
- Ensure child remains comfortable and reassure
- Ensure date and time of sample collection is written on request form and specimen
- Secure together and send to laboratory
- Record collection of sample in nursing documentation
- If sample is collected outside laboratory hours, place in a culture medium and store in specimen fridge.

Safety issues

- Care is needed when inserting tip of the swab into the nose, to avoid damaging the mucous membrane
- As young children may not co-operate, assistance will be required to prevent child moving during the procedure
- Gloves are worn for staff protection
- If patient is possibly infected with a high-risk organism, specimen and request form should be labelled with biohazard tape.

Adaptation for home care

- This procedure may be carried out in the home by community staff.

See *Appendix III*

Nursing notes

Nasogastric tube insertion (short term)

Definition: The insertion of a fine bore polyvinyl tube via the nose and oesophagus into the stomach

Purpose: To safely insert a nasogastric tube for artificial feeding and/or medication.

Equipment required

- Nasogastric tube. Selection of the correct size (width and length) will be dependent on child's age, size of nasal cavity and any anatomical considerations. As a guide, the following sizes are suggested:
  - ◆ Neonates FG 5–6
  - ◆ Toddlers FG 6–8 22 inch (56cm)
  - ◆ Older   FG 6–8 36 inch (91cm)
- Tape to mark and secure tube in place
- 50ml syringe
- Gallipot
- Sterile water to lubricate and flush nasogastric tube
- Blue litmus paper/pH paper
- Disposable gloves.

Psychological preparation and support

- Assess age and developmental level of infant/child
- Discuss pre and post-procedural preparation with play therapy department, to facilitate correct psychological preparation prior to incubation
- Assess child's and family's understanding of procedure
- Explain to child and family about the need for a nasogastric tube
- Rewards and stickers for the child can be used to promote confidence and self-esteem after the procedure. The rewards are not just for bravery but aim to give the message to the child that he/she attempted to master the difficult situation of having a tube passed and that it is appreciated, even if the child had difficulty complying. The reward emphasises that the child has endured the procedure
- Emphasis is placed upon the child and parent being in control as much as possible.

Nursing observations

- Check tube securely taped to restrict movement
- If there is uncertainty regarding correct positioning of tube, **reposition**
- Offer child a drink and aspirate stomach contents and test on litmus paper. If no acid reaction after reposition, tube again and contact medical staff. An x-ray may be required.

Nursing interventions

- Measure the length of nasogastric tube required. Place the distal end of tube at the tip of nose and extend the tube to the earlobe and down to the xiphoid process. Mark the length of tubing by placing tape on tube
- Ensure oxygen and suction is available
- Position the child appropriately. Infants are unresponsive; children should be placed in a supine position with head towards the side.
- Older children should be positioned in an upright position, maintaining a clear airway.

NB. Normal flexure of the cervical vertebrae tends to deflect the tube towards the trachea. Tilting the head back when the tube is moved beyond the nasopharynx increases this risk. Cervical flexure is lost when the head is flexed forward reducing the risk of tracheal intubation. The tongue and larynx move forward which tends to open the oropharynx and oesophagus respectively. This improves the change of oesophageal intubation. Excessive forward flexure inhibits swallowing.

- Wash hands and put on gloves
- Place the distal end of the tube in the water to lubricate the tip
- Encourage child to swallow while tube is inserted. Offer child/infant drink
- Gently insert the tube through the nose, directing it straight back along the floor of the nose
- Insert the tube posterially aiming the tip parallel to nasal septum and superior surface of hard palate
- Advance tube to nasopharynx, allowing tip to seek its own passage
- Insert the tube to be measured length. Observe for respiratory distress or inability to cry. Check tube position by aspirating sample of stomach contents
- As the child swallows advance the tube through oesophagus into stomach with a gentle motion.

NB. Coughing may indicate passage of tube into trachea. If this is suspected remove tube and reinsert. Particular care should be taken if any type of endotracheal device is in place or child has difficulty in swallowing, as it may tend to guide feeding tube into trachea.

- Check position of nasogastric tube by aspirating a sample of stomach contents. Test on litmus paper
- If a child is receiving antacids you will require the tube placement to be confirmed using aspirate on yellow pH litmus paper. The litmus paper should change colour to green. Use pH paper
- When tube is in correct position, secure tube to the side of face with tape. Mark tube with marker or tape to record tube position accurately. Document size of tube used, time, date of insertion, colour reaction of litmus paper and child's tolerance of procedure
- Using the above procedure, the nasogastric tube should be replaced weekly and this action documented
- Check surrounding skin during each span of duty to ensure skin remains intact
- Duoderm can be used underneath tape to prevent soreness.

Safety issues

- Irregularities in respiratory function, eg. excessive coughing. Remove the nasogastric tube and report immediately to medical staff
- If the child is distressed and refusing to co-operate, reassure and support the situation.

Adaptation for home care

- The principles of the procedure can be applied to the home care setting.

Further reading

Barnado LM, Bove MA (1993) *Paediatric Emergency Nursing Procedure.* Jones and Bartlett, London: 128–131

FACTSHEET Corflo Enteral feeding tubes Corpak Medsystems. Biomedical Lenten House, Lenton Street, Alton, Hampshire

Holden CE, MacDonald A, Ward M, Ford K *et al* (1997) Psychological preparation for nasogastric tube placement: psychological support. *British Journal of Nursing* **6**(7): 376–85

Metheny N (1988) Measures to test placement of nasogastric and nasointestinal feeding tubes. A Review. *Nursing Research* **37**(6): 324–9

Metheny N, Reed L, Wiersema L, McSweaney M *et al* (1993) Effectiveness of pH measurements in predicting feeding tube placement. An update. *Nursing Research* **42**(6): 324–31

Paul L, Holden C, Smith A *et al* (1993) *Tube Feeding and You*. Nutritional Care Department, The Birmingham Children's Hospital NHS Trust, Birmingham: 2–5

Sweeney SE (1982) Nasogastric tube care. In: Uroservich PR, Sapega SN, Obenrades MH (eds) *Performing Gastrointestinal Procedures*. Spring House, Pennsylvania: 44–70

Taylor S, Goodinson-McLaren S (1992) Enteral feeding equipment. In: *Nutritional Support: A Team Approach*. Wolfe Publishing Ltd, London

Welsh, JA, Dye JS, Games C, Ellett ML *et al* (1990). Staff nurses' experiences as co-investigators in a clinical research project. *Paediatric Nursing* **16**(4): 364–7

Young MH (1994) Preparation for nasogastric tube placement: Psychological support. In: Baker SB, Baker RD, Davis A (eds) *Paediatric Enteral Nutrition*. Chapman and Hall, London

See *Appendix III*

> *Nursing notes*

Nebulized solution, administration of

Definition: The administration of a nebulized solution

Purpose: This procedure can be used to moisten respiratory secretions, facilitate expectoration or suction, or be used to administer medication, eg. bronchodilators.

Equipment required

- Prescription chart/medication
- Medication
- 0.9% Sodium Chloride
- Compressed air/oxygen supply (as prescribed)
- Correct sized mask/mouthpiece and nebulizer chamber/s
- Tubing
- Tissues
- Secretions pot
- Medication
- Fg needle size 21
- 5ml syringe
- Saline
- Humidity may be beneficial if child has dry cough.

Nursing observations

- Observe child during procedure for compliance with administration
- Observe child and assess respiratory function prior to and following nebulizer, and record observations in nursing notes. This may include a Peak Flow recording
- Note any expectoration of respiratory secretions. Record observations in nursing notes as necessary and take specimens for laboratory analysis
- If the child has a poor response to nebulizer or demonstrates deterioration in respiratory function, record assessment in nursing notes and inform medical staff.

Nursing interventions

- Confirm child's identity bracelet against personal details on prescription chart
- Enable child to be positioned in a comfortable, relaxed position, sitting upright where possible
- Following local drug administration policy, place medication into nebulizer chamber and secure top/lid (see *Table 2.1*)
- Check medication literature to ascertain whether medication requires further dilution and at what pressure it should be delivered
- Attach nebulizer to air/oxygen supply
- Offer child, if able, opportunity to hold facemask/mouthpiece, or secure comfortably to child's face. This aspect of the procedure should ensure a seal around the mouth/nose to maximise inhalation of medication
- Switch on nebulizer and allow nebulizer to run until all the solution has been atomised, approximately ten minutes. NB. There may be some residual moisture in the chamber
- On completion, switch off nebulizer and remove all equipment from child's reach
- Cleanse nebulizer after each use and check for patency of equipment
- Store nebulizer and tubing in labelled paper bag with child's name. Change bag daily

- If child requires nebulizer for longer than seven-day period, sterilise the chamber once a week as per manufacturer's recommendations
- Assist and reassure child with expectoration of respiratory secretions as necessary
- Wash hands using Ayliffe Taylor method.

Table 2.1

Salbutamol (Ventolin ®)

The efficiency of a sulbutamol nebulizer is recognised to be dependant on the type of nebulizer used and the tolerance of the child to the procedure. Manufacturers acknowledge that there will be some residual volume remaining in the chamber

Preparations for salbutamol are usually presented as 2.5mg/5mg nebules in 2.5mls of sodium chloride. The pharmacy department advise further dilution to a volume of 4mls with additional sodium chloride prior to administration.

Ipratoropium Bromide (Atrovent ®)

The effect of Atrovent nebulisers is noted to be dependant on the type of nebulizer used. Nursing Staff are advised to follow the manufacturers guidelines for further dilution as necessary.

Safety issues

- Oxygen is often the delivery gas of choice if a child is in respiratory distress. However, the choice of carrier gas must be determined by child's clinical status
- If oxygen is used then it should be prescribed
- Compressed air is adequate for delivering routine or on-going treatment
- Inhalation technique: administering steroids may result in a rash over child's cheek
- Some evidence that children receiving long term steroids/ventolin/atrovent have increased incidence of glaucoma/cateracts. Care should be taken to avoid escape of inhalation from mask to child's eyes.

Adaptation for home care

The principles of the above procedure can be applied in the home. In addition, the following points should be checked:

- Smoking — advise carers that under no circumstances should smoking take place while nebulizer is being administered
- Ensure portable equipment is in safe working order and maintained in accordance with manufacturer's recommendations
- Ensure carers carry sufficient stocks of equipment to ensure portable use of nebulizer when necessary
- Advise carers if a child's condition deteriorates, to contact GP/Ambulance Service in first instance.

Discussion points

❖ Nebulized solution should ideally be finished within 10 minutes. A flow rate of at least 6–8 litres per minute of oxygen or air is required to achieve this.

❖ When nebulizing salbutamol, some degree of tremor and tachycardia may occur. Child/parents should be informed of this potential effect. This should be observed and reported to medical staff if severe

❖ Consider antifungal agent is prescribed as oral thrush is a common side effect of nebulized steroids.

Further reading

Clarke JE (1990) *Clinical Nursing Manual.* Prentice Hall, London

Owen J (1992) Asthma management pack national asthma campaign getting your breathing back. *Nursing Times* **88**(24): 70

Butler M (1998) Nebulisation: techniques and care. *Paediatric Nursing* **10**(9):17–20

British Medical Association (1998) *British National Formulary* **39**, March. BMA and Royal Pharmaceutical Society of Great Britain, London

See *Appendix III*

Nursing notes

Neurological observations

Definition: Observation of function of the central nervous system

Purpose: To access any neurological deficit following surgery or trauma of a child/infant.

Equipment required

- Pen torch/light source
- Neurological observation chart.

Psychological preparation and support

- Explain to family why you need to shine a bright light in both eyes
- Explain the reasons for the assessment as appropriate for age of child.

Nursing interventions

- Applying pressure on the side of the finger sufficient to evoke a response should create painful stimuli (avoid pressing on the nail bed)
- In specific circumstances it may be necessary to apply central stimuli (ie. supraorbital pressure)
- If there is a difference between right and left, score the best response
- If brain-stem, cervical spine cord or neuromuscular junction is impaired then the score is not applicable
- Score C if swelling or bandage closes eyes
- If no verbal (audible) response use grimace score
- Coma scale — best motor is the best arm response as there can often be spinal reflexes in the legs
- Record any significant events and number appropriately (see chart)
  - giving of sedative drugs
  - any fits noted
- It is often easier to see pupil reaction when overhead lighting is switched off.
- Neurological assessment is usually performed hourly
- Coma Score: add up numbered responses to arrive at a coma score
  - the lower the score the deeper the coma is
- Shine light into child's open eyes and wait for a few seconds to observe a pupil reaction.

Adaptation for home care

- Procedure remains the same — seek medical help if coma score worsening.

Further reading

Frawley P (1990) Neurological observations. *Nursing Times* **86**(35): 29–34

Tatman *et al* (1997) *Modified Paediatric Coma Scale* (adapted). Birmingham Children's Hospital NHS Trust, Birmingham

See *Appendix III*

Oral care using mouth swabs

Definition: A method of cleansing the mouth when tooth brushing is not tolerated or considered unsafe

Purpose: To cleanse and moisten the mouth, reduce plaque levels, reduce the likelihood of mouth infection and tooth decay.

Equipment required

- Clean tray, disposable/re-usable
- Disposable gloves
- Sterile gallipot
- Sterile water
- Chlorhexidine solution (or other, as prescribed)
- Foam mouth swabs or cotton buds, depending on the size of the child
- White soft paraffin for the lips.

Psychological preparation and support

- Explain procedure to child so he/she is prepared and to encourage co-operation.

Nursing observations

- Check mouth for signs of infection, ulcers, bleeding or loose teeth, before and throughout the procedure
- Observe for any gagging/choking or attempts to swallow cleansing fluid
- Check if the child's lips are dry and, if so, moisten them first for comfort.

Nursing interventions

- Cleanse the mouth twice daily with solution
- The same procedure using only water may be used between time to moisten the mouth
- Ensure child is comfortably positioned
- Wash hands
- Prepare equipment in clean tray
- Add chlorhexidine and/or water to the gallipot. Chlorhexidine strength should be 0.2% (if full strength chlorhexidine is not tolerated it may be diluted to half strength with water)
- Apply gloves
- Moisten swab well, but it should not be dripping
- Clean the teeth and gums with a circular action, starting at the back, as tolerated by the child
- Renew swab for each section, approximately five swabs used in all
- The cleaning motion should last for three minutes to be effective against plaque
- Ensure there is no pooling of fluid in the mouth
- Apply a pea-sized amount of white soft paraffin to the lips using sponge/bud or gloved finger.

Safety issues

- End or tip of swab or bud may, potentially, detach. If this happens ask the child to spit it out, otherwise use a gloved finger to 'sweep out' providing it is visible. If choking occurs, follow emergency guidelines for aspiration of a foreign body
- Use only water (not chlorhexidine) if sucking and swallowing is likely.

Adaptation for home care

- This procedure may be performed at home, when tooth brushing is not possible, following the same procedure
- Parents may choose not to wear gloves.

Discussion points

❖ Lip salve/lip balm may be preferred in place of white soft paraffin.

❖ Chlorhexidine should be prescribed in hospital. Full strength solution is best but if this is not tolerated it can be diluted to half strength with water.

Further reading

Ransier A, Ebstein J B, Lunn R, Spinell J (1995) A combined analysis of a toothbrush, foam brush, and chlorhexidine-soaked foam brush in maintaining oral hygiene. *Cancer Nursing* **18**(5): 393–6

Steelman R, Holmes D, Hamilton M (1996) Chlorhexidine spray effects on plaque accumulation in developmentally disabled patients. *Journal-Clinical-Paediatric-Dent* Summer **20**(4): 333–6

See *Appendix III*

Nursing notes

Oral care specific to oncology settings

Definition: Cleansing of mouth

Purpose: To reduce opportunistic infections while child is immunosuppressed. Specific oral care is needed for children receiving oncology treatment because of the alteration in the oral mucosa due to drug therapy.

Equipment required

- As for tooth brushing and oral care using mouth swabs procedure.

Psychological preparation and support

- Explain procedure to child so he/she is prepared and to encourage co-operation
- Mouth may be very sore, so a lot of reassurance that the procedure will help may be needed.

Nursing observations

- Mouth is formally examined once a day
- Check for signs of infection, ulcers, and bleeding or loose teeth
- Assess pain level prior to procedure and ensure analgesia is adequate
- Teaching of parents at the start of admission, so that they can be assessed as competent before discharge
- Oral care is performed four times a day, after main meals and before bed
- Use a soft toothbrush with toothpaste. Foam sponges or gauze swabs may be used as an alternative
- Corsadyl (chlorhexidine) mouthwash is used to rinse the mouth for 30–60 seconds, or can be applied with foam sponges. Oraldene mouthwash is used alternatively if Corsadyl is not tolerated
- Apply oral nystatin after tooth brushing and mouthwash, Fluconazole may be used as an alternative
- Child should have nothing to eat or drink for 10–15 minutes after mouthcare
- A local anaesthetic (eg. Difflam) may be prescribed for use ten minutes prior to procedure if mouth is painful
- Analgesia is often needed to control pain when mouth becomes sore, ulcerated and/or infected. (See *BCH Pain Management Protocol*, 1997.)

Safety issues

- If using mouth swabs or cotton buds, tip may potentially detach. If this happens, ask child to spit it out. Otherwise use a gloved finger to 'sweep out' provided it is visible. If choking occurs, follow emergency guidelines for aspiration of a foreign body
- Mouth wash solution is not to be swallowed – ensure child spits it out.

Adaptation for home care

- Oral care continues routinely at home as described while on course of oncology treatment.

Further reading

Beck SL (1992) *Prevention and Management of Oral Complications in the Cancer Patient.* JB Lippincott Company, Philadelphia

Galbraith I, Baily D, Kelly L, Rehn K *et al* (1991) Treatment for alteration oral mucosa related to chemotherapy. *Paediatric Nursing* **17**(3): 233–7

See *Appendix III*

Oral sedation

Definition: The administration of oral sedation and subsequent care

Purpose: To enable a child to remain still for a procedure without distress.

Equipment required

Equipment for giving sedation

- Prescription sheet
- Prescribed sedation
- Oral syringe, medicine pot or spoon
- Name band
- Drug formulary
- Drink (clear fluid only).

Equipment to have readily available

- Vomit bowl
- Oxygen supply
- Suction equipment
- Oxygen saturation monitor and probe
- IV cannulation equipment
- Guedal airway of appropriate size
- Access to resuscitation trolley.

Psychological preparation and support

- Discuss reasons for sedation with child and family and assess their understanding
- Explain procedure and need for monitoring to child and family to facilitate preparation and co-operation
- Explain side-effects of drugs with family and inform that after-effects may continue into the next day.

Nursing observations

- Prior to giving sedation record baseline observations; temperature, pulse, respiratory rate and effort, blood pressure oxygen saturation
- Check that any past or recent history of respiratory or nasopharyngeal problems has been medically assessed
- Nurse in an area where the patient is easily visible, with oxygen and suction available
- Maintain continuous pulse oximetry and check probe site after two hours for signs of trauma
- Record observations formally every quarter of an hour once the child is asleep (pulse, respiratory rate, rhythm, depth, sound and effort, and skin colour)
- If patient is being transferred to another department, hand over patient to a suitably qualified nurse or ODA. Nursing and medical notes to be complete and comprehensive, verbal report to be given.

Nursing interventions

- Patients having morning scan may have light early breakfast or patients having an afternoon scan may have light early lunch, both should exclude milk and eggs (breast milk excepted)
- Ensure sedation prescription is legible and within recognised dose ranges (local protocols exist and can be obtained from radiology department)

- Confirm patient details against prescription chart
- Give sedation following BCH oral drug administration procedure. Patient to be nil by mouth following administration
- Record administration
- Monitor effect of sedation
- If respiratory distress occurs, contact medical staff and commence appropriate emergency treatment as necessary, eg. maintain airway, give oxygen, suction if required, prepare for cannulation, insert guedal airway if necessary
- If agitation or confusion occurs, ensure that the immediate environment is safe, remove unnecessary equipment
- If vomiting occurs position patient to maintain clear airway. Do not repeat sedation without medical staff discussion
- If sedation fails (eg. child not asleep after 60 minutes) discuss with medical staff. IV sedation may be considered, but should only be administered in the presence of medical staff. Nursing responsibility for sedated patient continues
- Once successful sleep is achieved, continue with procedure for which sedation has been given, or telephone other department (eg. scanning) to let them know that patient is ready to be transferred
- Collect patient post procedure and receive verbal report, ensuring that patient is in stable condition for transfer
- Patient should stay in hospital until observations are stable and the child is awake and maintaining airway independently.

Safety issues

- Child should be assessed by medical staff on the day of sedation. Even slight colds may present airway problems once a child is sedated and not consciously protecting their airway
- Check resuscitation equipment/emergency support equipment is accessible and in good working order before commencing sedation
- Nurse patient in a bed/day case trolley in an uncluttered environment
- If patient is going to another department, transfer on a theatre or day case trolley with portable oxygen saturation monitor and guedal airway. They should not be carried by parents or transferred in pushchairs; refer to other relevant procedures, eg. oral medication, oxygen administration.

Best practice

❖ Suitability for sedation/exclusion criteria.

❖ Patients with known airway problems, eg. patients with nasopharyngeal tumors.

❖ Patients with cardiac/respiratory disease (cardiac patients may be considered if they are post surgery, off all cardiac drugs, and have approval of cardiologists)

❖ Patients with epilepsy (selected cases)

❖ Core care plans for sedated patients are available from Oncology/Haematology Day Care Unit.

Discussion point

❖ Great Ormond Street have a nurse-led Advanced Practice Sedation Team. They advocate 'sleep deprivation' as a factor in successful sedation, ie. parents are requested to keep the child up late, rise early and do not allow the child to sleep on the journey in. The 'crabbier' the child is on arrival the more likely they are to sedate easily.

Further reading

Having searched the literature for oral sedation/sedation protocols, there appears to be little information available except in the field of dental work.

See *Appendix III*

Nursing notes

Oxygen therapy

Definition: The administration of oxygen to correct hypoxia

Purpose: To oxygenate the child's arterial blood supply.

Equipment required

- Oxygen supply (portable/mains)
- Oxygen tubing
- Facemask/nasal speculae/nasal catheter/headbox
- Humidification system
- Oxygen saturation monitor
- Oxygen analyser if required
- Prescription chart.

Psychological preparation and support

- Discuss reasons for use of oxygen with child and family where possible and assess their understanding
- Explain procedure to child and family to facilitate preparation and co-operation.

Nursing observations

- Frequency of observations will be dependant on child's condition, not in relation to the need for oxygen
- Prior to commencing oxygen therapy record baseline observations of respiratory effort, eg. rate, rhythm, depth, evidence of sternal/abdominal recession, flaring of nostrils or tracheal tug and oxygen saturation
- Where an oxygen saturation probe is used, attach securely but not too tightly and ensure the site of attachment is checked every two to four hours to ensure that possible trauma, such as redness, blisters or lacerations do not occur
- Rotate site of probe as necessary
- Observe the child's response to oxygen therapy and record in nursing documentation.

Nursing interventions

- If there is poor patient response to delivery of oxygen increase oxygen flow, if prescribed, otherwise refer to medical staff
- Ensure prescription for oxygen therapy is legible and determines the concentration, method, and frequency of administration
- Prior to commencing oxygen therapy confirm the patient details against the prescription chart
- Commence oxygen therapy via chosen method
- Attach and secure oxygen saturation probe to chosen site on either fingers, toes or ear
- Record administration of oxygen – concentration, method and frequency in nursing documentation alongside an evaluation of the effect of oxygen therapy
- On commencement of oxygen therapy undertake hourly recording of respiratory rate and oxygen saturation levels and document
- Paediatric nurses may instigate/change oxygen therapy at their own initiative in critical situations. However, they must then ensure a medical review and subsequent written prescription at the earliest convenient time
- While child receives oxygen offer additional mouth care to maintain a moist mouth/lips to promote comfort

- Children do not tolerate face masks readily — ask them to hold the tubing and mask themselves or position close to their face to maximise the intake of oxygen. Where speculae or nasal catheter is used, taping to the face may reduce movement and irritation for child
- Where possible nurse child in a quiet environment
- If child is able to and interested, help select activities that can be undertaken without using much additional energy.

Safety issues

- Prescription of oxygen: oxygen is a drug and as such must be prescribed. Oxygen used in a paediatric setting must be monitored carefully to prevent damage to immature systems and delicate tissues
- Leak in system: check all components to reduce potential for leaks in system
- Where a child receives oxygen therapy it is essential that the level of oxygen delivered is measured through either a flowmeter or,in the case of children nursed in a headbox, an oxygen analyser. Ensure the analyser is recalibrated at commencement of each span of duty
- Oxygen is combustible therefore ensure that smoking is prohibited and equipment, that may spark, is not located near to a child receiving oxygen therapy.

Emergency use of oxygen

- Oxygen may be administered to a child in an emergency situation by registered nurses without a prescription.

Guidelines for the delivery of oxygen

- Nasal catheter/speculae
  - Use at flows < 3 litres/minute
  - May require humidification if prolonged use required
  - Ideal for post-operative oxygen therapy
  - Suitable particularly for neonates/infants
- Headbox
  - Use at flows > 4 litres/minute
  - Monitor oxygen concentration within headbox near to mouth/nose, using oxygen analyser
  - Humidity, required at high flows (> 7 litres/minute) and preferably warmed when used for prolonged periods
- Facemask
  - Use at flows > 3 litres/minute
  - Humidify at high flow ratc (> 5 litres/minute) or for prolonged use (> 6 hours)
  - Employ wide bore 'elephant' tubing for humidification
- Use of humidity
  - Humidity can be delivered by using either an:
    - AQUAPACK or INSPIRON

Best practice

Nasal catheter/speculae

❖ It is advised that the tubing is secured to the face to reduce movement and irritation. Position the tubing to the back of the head to reduce the risk of a strangulation hazard in infant/child.

Headbox

❖ Regularly wipe clean to remove condensation and reduce risk of cooling child/infant increasing their oxygen requirement.

Further reading

Wreck L, King EM, Dyer M (1986) *Illustrated Manual of Nursing Techniques.* 3rd edn. JB Lippincott Company, Philadelphia

See *Appendix III*

Nursing notes

Peak expiratory flow measurement

Definition: The measurement of the rate of airflow during forced exhalation, quantified in litres per minute

Purpose: To determine an accurate measurement of current respiratory function.

Equipment required

- Peak flow meter
- Correct size mouthpiece
- Child's nursing notes
- Black/red pen to document recordings.

Psychological preparation and support

- Assess age and development level of child/adolescent to facilitate correct preparation prior to procedure
- Assess child/adolescent's and family's understanding of procedure in order to reduce anxiety and facilitate co-operation
- Depending on age and development of child/adolescent they may have some difficulty in using peak flow meter. Whistles are available to attach which help child to recognise the correct technique
- Ensure child/family information is available in clinical area for further reference.

Nursing observations

- Assess child's general condition prior to undertaking procedure
- Do not attempt if respiratory state is too poor (see safety issues)
- Allow adequate rest between attempted recordings while observing the child for any deterioration/respiratory distress.

Nursing interventions

- Commence peak flow recordings as soon as possible following admission to hospital, if assessed safe to do so
- Measure and record the height of child/adolescent for use in monitoring ongoing relationship of height and lung function
- Following manufacturer's guidelines, prepare equipment for use
- Ask child/adolescent to stand upright where possible to maximise lung expansion
- Ask child/adolescent to inhale deeply and place mouthpiece in their mouth, ensuring the lips make a complete seal
- Ask the child/adolescent to blow forcefully into the peak flow meter as hard and as fast as possible
- Obtain a further two readings using the above method, allowing a period of rest in between each exhalation
- From the three recordings taken, note the highest reading and document in chart using a black pen
- If medication is prescribed, take a peak flow recording 30 minutes after administration to evaluate effect of medication
- Record pre-treatment recording in black and post-treatment recording in red
- Cleanse the peak flow meter according to manufacturer's instructions.

Safety issues

- Peak expiratory flow recordings should not be attempted on patients who have been identified as being in severe respiratory distress, however a poor reading from someone not previously identified as being in distress can be what alerts the nurse and medical staff to the degree of the problem
- Once this is identified, discontinue recordings until assessed safe to continue.

Adaptation for home care

- Procedure remains the same. Instruct child/parents to document highest of three recordings in community notes
- Advise parents to contact nursing/medical staff in the event of concern regarding low readings.

Discussion points

❖ A peak expiratory flow recording is only reliable as a measure of lung function when the child is proficient at performing the procedure.

❖ An acute asthma attack is not the time to teach any child the technique.

❖ Children under five years of age may not be able to comply sufficiently.

Further reading

Leach A (1994) Making sense of peak flow recordings of lung function. *Nursing Times* **90**(44): 34–5

Sharp J (1993) Which peak flow meter? *Nursing Times* **89**(3): 61–3

Seymour J (1995) Asthma. *Nursing Times* **91**(4): 50–2

Cartridge M (1990) *Guidelines for Health Professionals on the Measurement of Peak Flow*. National Asthma Campaign, London

Clement Clarke International Ltd (1993) *Peak Flow Measurement*. National Asthma Campaign, London

See *Appendix III*

Nursing notes

Platelets and granulocytes, collection and administration

Definition: Platelet sediment from platelet rich plasma, resuspended in 40–60ml plasma

Purpose: To treat thrombocytopenia.

Equipment required

- Prescription chart
- Identification form
- Administration set (platelets cannot be infused via a pump as the pump actions destroys the platelets.)
- Filter (will be stored with platelets).

Psychological preparation and support

- Assess age and developmental level of child/adolescent to facilitate preparation
- Consider whether religious observances may impact on the initiation of this treatment
- Filter (will be stored with platelets).

As per administration of blood. Refer to procedure number record administration of platelets in fluid balance chart/nursing records.

Nursing interventions

- For collection of platelets refer to procedure on blood product
- Platelets should be infused as a free infusion and not given via a pump
- Ensure a filter is always connected prior to commencing administration
- Platelets should be infused within 30 minutes of collection.

Safety issues

- Ensure correct patient identification against prescribed treatment
- Universal precautions — ensure correct procedures are followed when potentially coming into contact with bodily fluids
- Ensure batch numbers of all blood products administered are recorded in nursing/medical notes
- Dispose of used blood products in a separate 'sharps' box and keep in clinical area for 24 hours following administration
- Prior to disposal — ensure box labelled with patient name, registration number, and also ward/department name
- Blood product spillages — refer to Infection Control Policy Manual.

See *Appendix III*

Nursing notes

Pre-operative care

Definition: To prepare the infant/child and the family both physically and psychologically prior to any type of surgical procedure

Purpose: To reduce stress and ensure a safe delivery to theatre.

Equipment required

- Armband with accurate identification: name, age, date of birth, ward, and weight
- Allergies if identified on second armband
- Appropriate clothing
- Pre-operative Trust checklist.

Psychological preparation and support

- Explain procedure to child/parent/carer and allow time for questions to be asked
- Be sensitive to individual needs
- Previous experiences may influence the preparation and implementation of the procedure
- Consider age and development needs in preparing child and family
- Employ the play specialist skills as necessary
- Give encouragement and praise (bravery rewards/certificates).

Nursing observations

- Ensure Trust theatre checklist is accurate, completed and signed by a registered children's nurse prior to leaving the ward.

Nursing interventions

- Explain need for removal of outdoor clothing
- Check infant/child has fasted appropriately (intake of food six hours prior to anaesthesia, clear fluids two hours prior to anaesthesia)
- Record baseline observations of BP, pulse, temperature, respiration rate, height and urinalysis if appropriate
- Complete any specific medical instructions, eg. colonic washout, shave
- Complete Trust theatre checklist.

Adaptation for home care

- This procedure is not suitable for implementation at home.

Safety issues

- It is imperative that the child/adolescent wears an identification band. On arrival in theatre suite the accompanying nurse should raise any issues such as the presence of allergies, loose teeth etc. Any concerns should be addressed to the anaesthetic staff immediately on arrival in the department
- Opportunities to prepare a child prior to admission should be offered. This can include a visit to the ward, clinic, along with information pack.

Discussion points

❖ Depending on the age and development of the child they may have objections to wearing theatre gowns. If the child becomes distressed do not persist in trying to put gown on. Let child wear other clothes and contact theatres to let them know prior to transfer.

❖ Delays to the planned operating list can occur. Where a delay occurs consider the child who is nil by mouth. If the delay is to be substantial consider the need for intravenous fluids to be commenced.

❖ The Trust supports and encourages partnership in care. Where possible parents are encouraged to accompany their child to theatre. Due to pressure on available space, only one parent is encouraged to accompany the child to the anaesthetic room. If both parents wish to accompany the child it is advisable to contact the anaesthetist.

Further reading

Bagshaw O (1998) *Pre-operative Starvation Policy*. Birmingham Children's Hospital NHS Trust, Birmingham

See *Appendix III*

Nursing notes

Rectal washout

Definition: A method of cleaning the rectum using sterile fluid

Purpose: To remove faecal matter present in the rectum prior to diagnostic or surgical intervention.

Equipment required

- Rectal washout solution (warmed to 36–37°C)
- Protective undersheet
- Blankets/pillow
- Plastic apron and non-sterile gloves
- Lubricating jelly
- Gateclip/Spencer Wells forceps
- Funnel and tubing/20ml syringe
- Bucket (labelled with graduations)
- Correct sized rectal tubes (dependant on size of anus)
- Prescription chart.

Psychological preparation and support

- Depending on the child's age, understanding and developmental level this procedure may possibly be viewed as intrusive and the child may be uncooperative
- Explanation of all procedures prior to procedure being undertaken is essential to encourage a reduction in child anxiety and to maximise the child's cooperation
- Preparation prior to the procedure is essential to develop a sensitive rapport with the child prior to and during the procedure. Specialist help may be available from the Play Specialist
- Depending on the age and understanding of the child mild sedation may be prescribed prior to undertaking the procedure
- Due to the nature of the procedure it is essential that a quiet and private area be chosen to perform this procedure.

Nursing observations

- This procedure is potentially distressing and uncomfortable; it is therefore important to observe child's general well-being and level of anxiety. Giving support and reassurance as well as explaining each step of the procedure
- Prior to and following rectal washout the washout solution should be measured to ensure that none has remained in child's rectum leading to discomfort
- If after instilling fluid via the funnel on two occasions, no faecal matter/fluid is returned stop the procedure and inform medical staff
- If after repeated attempts fluid is heavily stained with faecal matter, stop procedure. It is better to undertake this procedure more frequently for shorter periods of time rather than for a very long time. This is essential to reduce local trauma and to aid patient comfort as the child can quickly cool down and become cold
- If after this approach the washout fluid continues to be heavily stained inform medical staff.

Nursing interventions

- Check child's identity band
- Administer prescribed oral sedation if necessary
- This procedure requires the assistance of two nurses (or a parent and nurse)

- Position infant/child on protective undersheet, ie. left lateral position, covering with a blanket
- Wash hands and apply gloves and an apron
- Attach funnel to tubing and connect to rectal catheter
- Lubricate the tip and first 1½ inches of rectal catheter with lubricating jelly
- Prime the rectal tubing with washout solution ensuring all air is expelled; clamp tubing
- Apply a generous smear of lubricating jelly to infant/child's anus
- Insert rectal catheter into rectum for 1½ inches, release clamp and allow fluid to run into bowel noting the amount of fluid used
- Invert and lower funnel and observe for return of fluid and faecal matter into bucket
- Repeat process of instilling fluid until fluid returned to bucket is clear
- In some circumstances the rectum may contain impacted faeces that will not be removed by the washout fluid alone. It is suggested that olive oil may be instilled into the rectum and child nursed in tilted bed to aid softening (infant 10mls/child 20mls)
- On completion of procedure assist child with repositioning and comfort
- Clear away all equipment
- Compare amount of fluid instilled and removed to ensure no surplus remains in rectum
- Wash hands using Ayliffe Taylor method.

Safety issues

- If the child is uncooperative enlist help of family and reward good behaviour
- Bleeding or pain during procedure: stop procedure. Inform medical staff. Keep child warm and record baseline observations of pulse, respiration and blood pressure
- If undertaking this procedure on a child between three and twelve years old, a 20ml syringe should be used as a funnel
- With all rectal washouts take care to stop procedure if no waste is expelled following two funnels of fluid being administered
- If child is known to have **CROHN's DISEASE** or **ULCERATIVE COLITIS** this procedure **should not be performed.** Bowel preparation can be implemented using the enteral route, reducing trauma locally in the bowel and for the child.

Adaptation for home care

- Procedure remains the same.

Adaptation for colostomy washout

- Procedure remains same, using correct size rectal catheter for stoma.

Adaptation for ileostomy washout

- It is not recommended that this procedure be undertaken without the direct written instructions of the child's consultant.

Discussion point

❖ Issues of praising for good behaviour: it is recommended to praise child for good behaviour and in this situation this might seem appropriate nursing behaviour. However, given the intimate nature of the procedure staff are advised not to use phrases such as 'good boy/girl' but to acknowledge that the procedure may be uncomfortable, but that it is nearly finished.

Further reading

Beck DE, Harford FJ, Palma JA (1985) Comparison of cleansing methods in preparation for colonic surgery. *Diseases of the Colon and Rectum* **28**(7): 491–5

Clarke B (1989) Bowel preparation for diagnostic procedures. *Nursing Times* **85**(5): 46–7

Ayliffe Taylor Handwash Technique

See *Appendix III*

Nursing notes

Recycling of stoma losses via distal stoma

Definition: The recycling of intestinal fluids

Purpose: To ensure the gut continues to function in the absence of nutrition.

Equipment required

- 5/10ml syringe
- 10cm lectrocath
- Syringe driver
- Feeding tube size 6 FG or 8 FG.

Psychological preparation and support

- Explain benefits to parents as part of the stoma care program.

Nursing observations

- Undertake routine recordings of temperature (core and skin), pulse and respiration every four hours
- Record all stoma fluid input and output from bowel actions on fluid balance chart
- Observe skin surrounding stoma for evidence of redness/excoriation
- Check site every two to four hours to ensure patency of feeding tube.

Nursing interventions

- Collect ileostomy or jejunostomy fluids from stoma bag
- Draw up stoma fluids with syringe and attach to lectrocath and prime line expelling any air
- Attach lectrocath to feeding tube
- Connect syringe to syringe driver and set driver to instil stoma fluids over four hours
- Repeat procedure as necessary.

Safety issues

- Establish integrity of lower bowel prior to commencing procedure
- Observe for signs of perforation.

Complications

- Intestinal obstruction
- Perforation of bowel
- Leakage of effluent over child's skin/stoma site.

Adaptation for home care

- This procedure is not suitable for implementation at home.

See *Appendix III*

Reverse barrier nursing (protective isolation)

Definition: The protection of immuno-comprised patients from acquiring an infection

Purpose: To reduce the potential of a sick child acquiring an infection while in hospital.

Equipment required

- Single clean room is essential (with negative pressure ventilation if available). Refer to Infection Control Policy — Section F
- White Isolation Card
- Outside the room access to handwash facilities and alcohol rub
- Plastic aprons and disposable gloves.

Psychological preparation and support

- Explain to child and family the need for care to be delivered in isolation
- Liaise with play specialist to ensure appropriate play/activities are available
- Consider needs of child who is isolated from others and adapt care.

Nursing observations

- Ensure all visitors to ward comply with Infection Control Policy.

Nursing interventions

- VISITORS: ensure all report to the nurse in charge or named nurse of child/adolescent before entering the room (refer to policy for Prevention of Transmission of Infection to and from Hospital Visitors — Section C)
- Restrict visitors to close family if necessary
- Identify key nursing staff to be involved in child's/adolescent's care
- Prior to entering room wash hands
- On entering room
    - put on an apron
    - use alcohol rub
    - put on gloves
    - perform specific nursing interventions as necessary
- Dispose of soiled linen and rubbish/clinical waste as per Infection Control Policy
- Remove apron/gloves inside cubicle and wash hands
- During the period of protective isolation ensure the child's social and psychological needs are met through appropriate use of play, activities or entertainment
- Explain and ensure child and family are aware of the nurse call system
- Liaise with play specialist team/teachers in delivery of care.

Safety issues

- Keep harmful equipment/hazards out of reach to children
- Daily cleansing of room should be supervised in accordance with guidelines in the Infection Control Policy
- Should the child need to leave the unit, relevant information regarding isolation procedures should be forwarded to the relevant head of department.

Adaptation for home care

- The principles of this procedure can be applied in the home, although strict protective isolation does not apply.

Further reading

The Royal College of Nursing (1994) *Guidance on Infection Control in Hospitals*. RCN, London
Bowell B (1992) Hands up for cleanliness. *Nursing Standard* **6**(15/16): 24–5

See *Appendix III*

Nursing notes

Routine tooth brushing

Definition: Cleansing of the mouth daily using a toothbrush

Purpose: To cleanse the mouth, reduce plaque levels, reduce the likelihood of mouth infection and tooth decay.

Equipment required

- A soft toothbrush with a small head, for individual child's use
- Use child's own toothbrush (if it is in a suitable condition), particularly if they have a specifically adapted one
- A pea-sized amount of fluoride toothpaste or children's toothpaste
- Disposable gloves if contact with oral secretions are likely.

Psychological preparation and support

- Tooth brushing should start when the baby's first teeth appear
- All children under seven years of age should be assisted with tooth brushing
- Children over the age of seven who are ill or disabled may need assistance
- Prepare the child by explaining what is going to happen
- If the child wishes to 'have a go' at brushing his/her own teeth first, this should be encouraged.

Nursing observations

- Check mouth for signs of infection, ulcers, bleeding or loose teeth, before and throughout the procedure
- Observe for any gagging/choking or attempts to swallow cleansing fluid
- Check if the child's lips are dry and, if so, moisten them first for comfort.

Nursing interventions

- Teeth should be brushed twice a day, in the morning and before bed
- Put toothpaste onto brush
- To assist the child, stand behind and tilt their head back. Then clean the teeth with a gentle circular or backward and forward motion
- A taller child or someone unable to stand, may sit in a chair or on a beanbag
- To assist someone lying in bed, brush one side of the mouth at a time, first the upper teeth and then the lower
- Brushing the teeth should include brushing the gum area
- To be fully effective, tooth brushing should take three minutes
- Child should spit out after brushing but does not have to rinse the mouth
- Suctioning can be used to remove froth and secretions from the mouth
- Remove toothpaste from around mouth
- A healthy, well balanced diet is an important part of oral health. Sugar intake should be controlled (sugar should not be in contact with the teeth for extended lengths of time)
- Six-monthly dental checks are advised for long-stay patients, from the time that the first teeth appear.

Safety issues

- Seek medical advice if ulcers, bleeding or infection are seen in the mouth
- Adult toothpaste is not meant to be swallowed — switch to a child's brand if this is a problem
- If child can only be flat, or is prone to choking, ensure suction is at hand
- Consider the use of mouth swabs if tooth brushing is painful or difficult.

Adaptation for home care

- Procedure remains the same.

Discussion points

❖ There is some disagreement about whether children should use fluoride toothpaste in areas where fluoridation of the water is common, eg. West Midlands. An excess of fluoride can lead to flucrosis and a child's second set of teeth can be damaged due to an excess of fluoride. Children and parents should be advised to ensure that children do not swallow excess toothpaste.

❖ Controversy surrounds the techniques to correct brushing; single strokes away from the gums or a continuous circular action having both been advocated. At this time no one method appears preferable to teach children. However, the child should be encouraged to brush their teeth routinely to promote oral health.

Further reading

Kite K, Pearson L (1995) A rationale for mouth care: the integration of theory with practice. *Intensive Care and Critical Care Nursing* **11**(2): 71–6

Pearson LS (1996) A comparison of the ability of foam swabs and toothbrushes to remove dental plaque; implications for nursing practice. *Journal of Advanced Nursing* **23**(1): 62–9

General Dental Council and British Society of Dentistry for the Handicapped and the British Paedodontric Society (1997) *Healthy Mouth, Happy Smile* booklet.

Health Education Authority (1997) *Looking after your mouth.* HEA, London

Health Education Authority (1997) *Keeping baby teeth healthy — tooth care for 0–2 year olds.* HEA, London

Health Education Authority (1997) *Caring for your children's teeth — tooth care for 3–11 year olds.* HEA, London

See *Appendix III*

Nursing notes

Scar massage

Definition: The massage of scar tissue

Purpose: To improve the long term appearance of a scar.

Equipment required

- E45 or Nivea cream/lanolin.

Psychological preparation and support

- Explain to child and parents reasons for performing procedure
- Explain to child that procedure is not painful.

Nursing observations

- Ensure that scar tissue and surrounding skin is intact before commencing. Do not proceed if skin is sore, broken or inflamed.

Nursing intervention

- Apply cream to scar
- Use firm circular movements with fingers to massage scar for five minutes.

Safety issues

- Nurses to wear gloves when performing procedure
- Handwashing before and afterwards
- Do not perform on broken or infected skin
- Wound should be at least 14 days old.

Adaptation for home care

- Advise child and parents to carry out procedure two to four times a day for three months.

See *Appendix III*

Nursing notes

Silk nasogastric tube

Definition: Insertion of a fine bore nasogastric tube via the nose and oesophagus into the stomach

Purpose: To introduce the correct type of tube for providing nutritional support/medication directly into the stomach.

Equipment required

- Polyurethane tube (silk)
- Selection of the correct size (width and length) will be dependent on child's age, size of nasal cavity and any anatomical considerations. The type of feed to be delivered and the method used to deliver the feed. As a guide, the following sizes are suggested:
  - Neonates FG 5–6
  - Toddlers FG 6–8 22 inch (56cm)
  - Older   FG 6–8 36 inch (91cm)
- Sterile water to flush tube
- 50ml syringe
- Gallipot
- Litmus paper/pH paper
- Tape to mark and secure tube
- Unsterile gloves.

Psychological preparation and support

- Assess age and developmental level of infant/child
- Discuss pre- and post-procedural support with play therapy department. To facilitate correct psychological preparation prior to intubation
- Assess child's and family's understanding of the procedure
- Explanation to child and family about the need for a nasogastric tube
- Rewards and stickers for the child can be used to promote confidence and self-esteem after the procedure. The rewards are not just for bravery but aim to give the message to the child that he/she has attempted to master the difficult situation of having a tube passed and that this is appreciated: even if the child has difficulty in complying the reward emphasises that the child has endured the procedure. Emphasis is placed upon the child and parent being in control as much as possible.

Nursing observations

- If the tube will not flush then the tube is probably blocked. Gently put 5mls of air down the tube. Aspirate tube to check patency of tube. If no aspirate is obtained, discontinue use of tube. Inform senior nursing staff. Reposition tube if necessary.

Nursing interventions

- Remove tubes and guide wire from package. Prior to insertion of tube, flush tube with 2–3mls of water. Check that the guide wire moves freely. Do not use the guide if it is bent
- Thread the guide wire down the tube and ensure the guide wire is securely in position
- Measure the length of tube to be inserted to assume that the tip enters the fundus of the stomach. Place the distal end of tube at the tip of nose and extend the tube to the earlobe and down to the xiphoid process in the infant. The tubes should be positioned midway between umbilicus and xipisternum. Mark the tubing at the required length using tape
- Ensure oxygen and suction is readily available during procedure

- Position child for nasogastric tube insertion. Infants and unresponsive children in a supine position. For older children place in an upright position. Ensure airway is patent.

NB. Normal flexure of the cervical vertebrae tends to deflect the tube towards the trachea. Tilting the head back when the tube is moved beyond the nasopharynx increases this risk. Cervical flexure is lost when the head is flexed forward reducing the risk of tracheal intubation. The tongue and larynx move forward which tends to open the oropharynx and oesophagus respectively. This improves the change of oesophageal intubation. Excessive forward flexure inhibits swallowing.

- Wash hands and put on gloves (universal precautions)
- Place the end of the tube in the water to lubricate the tip. Facilitates tube insertion
- Encourage child to swallow while tube is being inserted
- Offer a drink by cup or bottle as appropriate.
- Insert the tube posterially aiming tip parallel to nasal setum and superior surface of hard palate
- Insert the tube to the measured length. Observe for respiratory distress or inability to cry. Check position of nasogastric tube by aspirating a sample of stomach contents
- Advance tube to nasopharynx, allowing tip to seek its own passage. As the child swallows, with a gentle motion advance the tube through the oesophagus into stomach.

NB: Coughing may indicate passage of tube into trachea. If suspected, remove tube and reinsert. Particular care should be taken if any type of endotracheal device is in place, or child has difficulty in swallowing as it may tend to guide feeding tube into trachea.

- Aspirate 4–5mls and test the content on a sample of litmus paper. This should change colour to pink
- If a child is receiving antacids please use pH paper; yellow paper must change to green (1–6pH). Document in nursing notes colour reaction pH
- Secure tube to the side of the face with tape as appropriate. Mark tube of nostril to ensure tube does not move. Document time, size of tube used and date of insertion. Record nursing intervention and give information on when tube next needs to be replaced. Mark tube by nostril with tape or marker pen to identify tube position accurately
- Flush tube with 5mls of water using a 50ml syringe. (NB. Smaller syringes exert higher pressures to the tube walls leading to possible tube damage)
- The tube should be flushed at least three times each day to prevent blockage, ie.
  - prior to commencing a feed
  - following discontinuation of a feed
  - before and after giving medicines
- Using the above procedure the nasogastric tube should be placed monthly and this action documented.

Safety issues

- Unable to aspirate from nasogastric tube
- When checking for placement of aspiration withdraw syringe plunger slowly. If it is difficult to obtain a gastric aspirate, distal tip of tube may be above fluid level in stomach .To overcome this, offer child a drink, place child on left side, wait a few minutes for tube tip to fill below fluid level. Attempt aspiration of gastric contents again
- Tube may need to be repositioned, x-ray may be taken to assess tube position if problems persist

- Irregularities in respiratory function, eg. excessive coughing
- Remove the nasogastric tube and report immediately to medical staff
- Child is distressed and refusing to cooperate: reassure and support the child during the process of having a tube passed.

See *Appendix I* for further guidance on tube placement

Adaptation for home care

- The principles of the above procedure can be applied in the home setting.

Further reading

Barnado LM, Bove MA (1993) *Paediatric Emergency Nursing Procedure.* Jones & Bartlett, London: 128–31

Holden CE, MacDonald A, Ward M, Ford K *et al* (1997) Psychological preparation for nasogastric tube placement: Psychological support. *British Journal of Nursing* **6**(7): 376–85

Paul L, Holden C, Smith A *et al* (1993) *Tube Feeding and You.* Nutritional Care Department, The Birmingham Children's Hospital NHS Trust, Birmingham: 5

Metheny N (1988) Measures to test placement of nasogastric and nasointestinal feeding tubes. A review. *Nursing Research* **37**(6): 324–9

Metheny N, Reed L, Wiersema L, McSweaney M *et al* (1993) Effectiveness of pH measurements in predicting feeding tube placement. An update. *Nursing Research* **42**(6): 324–31

Sweaney SE (1982) Nasogastric tube care. In: Uroservich P, Sapega SN, Obenrades MH (eds) *Performing Gastrointestinal Procedures.* Intermed Communication Inc, Springhouse, Pennsylvania: 44–70

Taylor S, Goodinson-McLaren S (1992) Enteral feeding equipment. In: *Nutritional Support: A team approach.* Wolfe Publishing Ltd, London: Ch 9

Young MH (1994) Preparation for nasogastric tube placement: Psychological support. In: Baker SB, Baker RD, Davis A (eds) *Paediatric Enteral Nutrition.* Chapman and Hall, London

FACTSHEET *Corflo Enteral Feeding Tube.* Corpak Medsystems Biomedical Lenten House, Lenton Street, Alton, Hampshire

See *Appendix III*

Nursing notes

Suction

Definition: To clear the upper airways of secretions with a suction catheter and vacuum pump

Purpose: To avoid retention of secretions in a child/infant who is unable to cough effectively, or to maintain a patient's airway.

Equipment required

- Suction catheters
- Single sterile disposable gloves
- Suction tubing
- Vacuum pump.

NB. Suction tubing should be changed daily and suction contents disposed of in a sealed container.

Psychological preparation and support

- Appropriate explanation of procedure for the age of the child.

Nursing observations

Suction should never be done routinely but only as required.
- Suction can cause hypoxia, therefore oxygen should be available during the procedure
- Introduction of saline into endotracheal tube prior to suctioning is a technique of debatable effectiveness but does include coughing.

Adverse effects of suction
- Mucosal trauma
- Hypoxia
- Emotional distress to parent or child
- Increased blood pressure
- Vagal stimulation
- Pneumothorax
- Atelectasis
- Cardiac arrest
- Discomfort
- Intra-ventricular haemorrhage in pre-term babies
- Tachycardia
- Apnoea
- Increased bronchospasm
- Arrhythmias and damage to any incisions
- Infection.

NB. A child should only be disconnected from a ventilator for the minimum amount of time.

Nursing interventions

- Wash hands using Ayliffe Taylor method
- Prepare a clean surface to open suction catheters onto
- Open end of appropriately sized suction catheter packaging so that coloured end is visible (see chart opposite)
- Put on sterile disposable glove on dominant hand

- Attach suction catheter to suction tubing maintaining aseptic technique
- Switch on vacuum pump to appropriate pressure (see below)
- Commence suction procedure
  - Endotracheal: pass suction catheter down endotracheal tube until resistance is felt
  - Nasal: Pass suction catheter into nasopharynx until a cough is inhaled
    - neonates — upper airway suction only
  - Oropharynx: use an appropriate sized yankeur sucker, if able
- Apply negative suction pressure only on exit
- Use continuous rather than intermittent suction ensuring that suction pressure goes no higher than 20 Kpa in baby/neonate, 25 Kpa in a child and 30 Kpa in a teenager/adolescent
- After completion of procedure, clear away rubbish, wash hands using Ayliffe Talor method and document amount, consistency and colour of secretions.

Suction pressure

60–120mmHg/8–16 Kpa in infants and children

Pressure should not exceed 150mmHg/20 Kpa in adults

Suction catheter size

(French gauze)		
	5–6 FG	Neonates
	6–8 FG	Babies
Oral/nasal	8 FG	Infants and young children
	10FG	Large children and adolescents
	12 FG	Adults
Endotracheal	4.0 ETT	Size 6–8 FG
	3.5 ETT	Size 6–7.5 FG
	8.0 ETT	Size 10FG–14FG
	Over 8.0 ETT	Size 14 FG + Over

If endotracheal tube is blocked, use largest size catheter that you can safely put down.

Further reading

Brazier D (1999) Endotracheal Suction Technique – putting research into practice. *Journal of Associates of Chartered Physiotherapy in Respiratory Care* **32**: 13–17

Lovatt May S (1993) *Teaching Package on Endotracheal Suctioning.* Intensive Care Unit, Birmingham Children's Hospital NHS Trust, Birmingham

Macmillan C (1995) Nasopharyngeal suction study reveals knowledge deficit. *Nursing Times* 13 December **91**(50)

See *Appendix III*

Suppository/enema, administration of

Definition: The administration of prescribed medication via the rectum

Purpose: To promote absorption of medication via the rectal mucous membrane or to assist in emptying of the rectum.

Equipment required

- Prescribed medication
- Disposable gloves
- Tissues
- Protective undersheet and blanket
- Lubricating jelly/water
- Toilet facilities as necessary, eg. bedpan, commode.

Psychological preparation and support

- Prior to procedure explain to child and family purpose and nature of intervention to reduce anxiety and promote co-operation
- Ensure child and family understand whether procedure will have medicinal/clearance effect
- Consider when would be the most appropriate time to perform procedure, ensuring privacy at all times.

Nursing observations

- Observe child during procedure and give continuing reassurance as necessary
- Observe and record effect of procedure and results.

Nursing interventions

- Explain procedure appropriate to child's age and developmental level involving family
- Select a private/quiet area of ward to undertake procedure
- Explain to child and parent/carer the drug being given and why, how it is administered and any possible side-effects
- Check medication against prescription chart and calculate required dosage
- Prepare bed area with undersheet
- Lubricate suppository/enema according to manufacturer's instructions
- Position child on left side with knees drawn up
- Put on gloves and insert suppository into rectum (round end first) beyond the anal sphincter
- If administering an enema, ensure fluid is warmed to body temperature before administration
- If the purpose of medication is to empty the rectum give child and family information on how long to retain medication and positioning, as well as where the nearest toilet facilities are available
- If medication is for analgesic properties explain this clearly and gain the child's and/or family's consent to proceed.

Safety issues

- Ensure clear explanations are given to both child and parent regarding the choice of method for administration of medication.

Insertion into a stoma/colostomy

- In some cases the child may have an anal anomaly resulting in no rectal opening. The procedure may be performed in the same manner as per rectum.

Adaptation for home care

- Procedure may be undertaken in the home as stated.

Discussion points

❖ Concern may be expressed by parents/child regarding the method of administration, particularly in view of the issue of child abuse.

❖ Encourage child/parents to express any concerns.

❖ Ensure that they have full understanding of the reasons for method being chosen, eg. absorption rates.

❖ Gain the child and family's consent.

❖ Recent writings suggest that using water to lubricate suppositories rather than a jelly lubricant reduces the time taken for the suppository to be absorbed and so enhances its effectiveness.

❖ Giving praise to children is an important aspect of nursing care particularly when a child is involved in an uncomfortable procedure. However, given the nature of this procedure care should be taken to consider how praise might potentially be received by children. It may be more appropriate to consider whether praise is appropriate in this situation as evidence from child abuse studies show that this element of trust can be abused by those in authority or responsible for a child's care. An alternative approach might be to acknowledge that the procedure would be uncomfortable but that it will not take long and that the child will be able to resume their usual activities shortly afterwards.

Further reading

Wieck L, King EM, Dyer M (1986) *Illustrated Manual of Nursing Techniques*. 3rd edn. Lippincott, Philadelphia: Ch 100

Whaley L, Wong D (1993) *Nursing Care of Infants and Children*. 4th edn. Mosby, St Louis,

Smith D (1991) *Comprehensive Child and Family Nursing Skills*. Mosby, St Louis

See *Appendix III*

Nursing notes

Temperature, pulse and respiratory rate, the taking of

Definition: Temperature   The balance between heat production and heat loss.

Pulse   The local rhythmic expansion of an artery, which can be felt with the finger, corresponding to each contraction of the left ventricle of the heart.

Respiration   The gaseous interchange between the tissue cells and the atmosphere.

Purpose: To obtain baseline vital signs. For early detection of deviation from the normal limits/deterioration in condition.

Equipment required

- Watch with second hand
- Appropriate chart to record results
- Thermometer (glass/disposable/electronic)
- Disposable sheath/cleaning agent — steret, tissue
- Lubricating jelly if using rectal route for temperature.

Psychological preparation and support

- Explain the procedure to the child and family in an age appropriate way, relevant to their understanding
- Rectal temperatures can be distressing/embarrassing for older children and are generally not appropriate for this age group
- Involve parents in taking observations — ensure they inform staff of their findings
- Temperature, pulse and respiration observations are likely to be more accurate if the child and family are relaxed.

Nursing observations

- Note any deviation from baseline observation or deviation from normal limits. Report to medical staff if deviation persists
- Note normal limits of pulse and respiration to specific age groups
- Observe recommendations produced by manufacturers for devices for taking temperature
- Be aware that pulse and respiration rate can alter if the child is in pain/discomfort
- Note the temperature of the environment as it can have dramatic effects on young children whose temperature control is immature
- Sick children require rest — continual disturbances can distress them, do other caring procedures at the same time to reduce disruption.

Nursing interventions

- Discuss relevance of taking observations with the child and family prior to carrying out the procedure, taking into account the child's age, developmental level and physical condition
- Take in the following order — respiratory rate , pulse and then temperature. This increases the co-operation and produces more accurate results as the least intrusive procedure is done first.

Respiration

- Be in view of the child's abdomen/chest to assess respiratory status, the child may or may not be aware that you are assessing him/her
- Ensure the child is at rest, as activity can dramatically increase the child's respiratory rate

- Count the rate of respiration's for one minute (do not count rate for less than one minute as a child's respiratory rate can alter quickly over a short period of time)
- Observe for recession (intercostal/tracheal), nasal flaring, cyanosis (lips/nose/ear lobes), and audible expiratory wheeze as this could indicate respiratory distress. Report to medical staff if observed
- Record on appropriate chart running notes; observe for deviations from previous respiratory rate pattern.

Pulse

- Decide which site the pulse is to be taken — radial, brachial, pedal or temporal
- Locate pulse with index finger — and count rate for one minute, observing for rhythm and strength
- If any deviations/abnormalities persist report to medical staff.

Temperature

- Assess which route/tool is most desirable, taking into account the child's age/developmental level (rectal temperature favourable for a child one year and under except any child with an acute abdomen, blood in stools or nappy, or suspected of having NEC (Necrotizing Entorocolotis)
- Ensure the thermometer is clean/covered with a disposable sheath and at the minimum reading
- **Axilla**: position the thermometer under the child's arm ensuring the two skin surfaces are touching around the thermometer for a minimum of five minutes
- **Oral**: position the thermometer into the child's mouth under the tongue (ensure the child's understanding of possible dangers) for a minimum of three minutes
- **Inguinal**: position the thermometer between the two skin surfaces for a minimum of five minutes
- **Rectal**: lubricate the thermometer and insert bulb end 1–1½cm into the child's rectum for a minimum of two minutes
- Remove the thermometer and determine the temperature, and record on an appropriate chart
- Report deviations in excess of normal temperature limits, ie. 37°C to medical staff; dress child appropriately and give anti-pyretics as prescribed
- **Tympanic**: Follow manufacturer's instructions
- **Tempdots**: Apply strip to stain and follow manufacturer's instruction.

Safety issues

- Be aware that carotid artery can be occluded with young children
- Do not take oral temperatures on young children, especially if using a glass thermometer, as there is risk of breakage and a hazard to child's health
- Beware of doing rectal temperature (necessary for children who are peripherally shut down) if the child has abnormalities with their gastric intestinal tract
- Depends on a child's condition — broken limbs etc — where pulse can be taken
- Be aware of trauma to the bowel resulting in perforation of the bowel.

Adaptation for home care

- Temperature, pulse and respiration can be observed in the same way as already discussed.

Further reading

Haddock BJ, Merrow DL, Swanson MS (1996) The Falling Grace of Axillary Temperatures. *Paediatric Nursing* **22**(2): 121–5

Board M (1995) Comparison of disposable and glass mercury thermometers. Royal Bournemouth Hospital. *Nursing Times* **91**(33): 36–7

Pontious S, Kennedy AH, Shelley S, Mittrucker C (1994) Accuracy and reliability of a temperature measurement by instrument and site. *Journal of Paediatric Nursing, Nursing Care of Children and Families* **9**(2): 114–23

Pontrais S, Kennedy A, Chung KL, Burroughs TE *et al* (1994) Accuracy and reliability of temperature measurement in the emergency department by instrument and site in children. *Paediatric Nursing* **20**(1): 58–63

Whaley L, Wong D (1983) *Nursing Care of Infants and Children.* Mosby, St Louis

Burke K (1996) Education. The tympanic membrane thermometer in paediatrics: a review of the literature. *Accident and Emergency Nursing* **4**(4): 190–3

Weller F, Wells J (1990) *Baillière's Nurses Dictionary, 21st Edition.* Baillière Tindall, London

See *Appendix III*

> *Nursing notes*

Throat swab collection

Definition: The collection of a sample of oro-pharyngeal secretions for the purpose of laboratory examination

Purpose: To obtain a specimen for laboratory study to determine the presence and specific type of a micro-organism.

Equipment required

- Dry sterile specimen swab
- Culture medium, for use if swab is not sent to laboratory immediately
- Request form
- Vomit bowl and tissues
- Clean spatula, if required
- Disposable gloves
- Pen torch.

Psychological preparation and support

- Consider child's age and understanding when preparing for procedure. Involve the parents if available
- Assess the physical condition of the child when planning the method (positioning) to be used.

Nursing observations

- Consider child's routine when planning to undertake procedure, avoid after food or drink has been taken, to reduce the chances of vomiting
- Observe the mouth during procedure for any obvious signs of thrush, ulcers, bleeding, swelling, or pus. If pus is evident in the throat, the sample collected should include this
- Observe for gagging or choking and be alert for possibility of vomiting during sample collection.

Nursing interventions

- Explain procedure to child and parents/carers
- Check child's identity against request
- Prepare equipment
- Label swab container with child's name, registration number and ward
- Position child in an upright position if possible, or an alternative safe position, in a well-lit area
- Wash hands using Ayliffe Taylor method
- Put on gloves
- Encourage child to open mouth wide
- Stroke the cheeks, or gently compress both sides of the jaw if child unable to comply
- Ask child to say 'aah' to enable insertion of swab to the back of the mouth
- If child cannot assist with 'aah' a spatula may be carefully used to depress tongue
- A pen torch may be required to give light to back of mouth
- Rotate swab around oro-pharynx, particularly around the tonsil bed
- Withdraw the swab, taking care to avoid touching any other part of the mouth
- Carefully place the swab in the designated container and seal
- Dispose of gloves and spatula

- Reassure child, re-positioning comfortably
- Wash hands and dry hands thoroughly
- Ensure date and time of sample collection is written on request form and specimen
- Attach together and send to laboratory
- Record collection of sample in nursing documentation
- If sample is collected outside laboratory hours, place in a culture medium and store in specimen fridge.

Safety issues

- **This procedure must not be attempted if epiglottitis is suspected, as an airway obstruction is likely to result**
- If there is a high risk of vomiting during the procedure then the position selected must allow ready drainage of vomit. Ensure suction apparatus is available
- Care is needed when inserting the spatula or specimen swab in the mouth to avoid damaging the oral mucosa
- Gloves are worn in accordance with universal precautions
- If patient is possibly infected with a high-risk organism, specimen and request form should be labelled with biohazard tape.

Adaptation for home care

- This procedure is not normally carried out at home, but may be performed by community staff. Portable suction must be available.

Discussion point

❖ Consider the rights of the child and the consent of the parents/carers if exerting pressure to open the mouth.

See *Appendix III*

> *Nursing notes*

Topical anaesthetic

Definition: Application of local anaesthetic for diagnostic or therapeutic interventions

Purpose: To reduce localised pain and trauma.

Equipment required

- Anaesthetic cream of choice, eg. EMLA, Ametop
- Occlusive dressing, eg. Opsite, Tegaderm
- Cotton bandage if required
- Tape to secure bandage
- Prescription chart.

Psychological preparation and support

- Explain procedure to child/parents, allowing time for questions
- Be sensitive to individual needs as previous experiences may influence the preparation and implementation of the procedure (consider age and developmental needs)
- Employ the play specialist skills as necessary
- Give a reward from the reward box, eg. certificate or badge/toy for bravery.

Nursing observations

- Identify suitable sites for application, avoiding broken skin
- Observe skin for signs of a reaction following application
- Involve parents in monitoring security of dressing.

Nursing interventions

- Check expiry date of chosen cream and read instructions for application
- Identify correct patient/child/infant against prescription chart
- Identify suitable cannulation sites — medical staff to identify specific sites as necessary
- Ensure hand site is clean and dry
- Apply half the contents of tube on identified site
- Cover cream with occlusive dressing
- Apply bandage as necessary over occlusive dressing depending on child's age
- After identified time, remove cream as per instructions given by the manufacturer and record time in nursing notes
- Mark sites on removal of cream.

Safety issues

- Check child for known allergies as application of local anaesthetic cream may result in an allergic reaction
- Document the time of application and removal in nursing notes.

Discussion points

EMLA cream

❖ Eutectic mixture of local anaesthetics.

❖ Action: acts by vasoconstriction on capillaries.

Application

❖ Not to be used on children under one year of age.

❖ Apply cream for a minimum of 60 minutes, to a maximum of five hours. (Efficacy may decline if left longer.)

❖ Avoid contact with eyes, mouth and mucosal surfaces.

Removal

❖ Site must be assessed immediately for venepuncture once cream has been removed.

❖ Observe skin condition following procedure and note any reactions and record in the nursing notes and inform medical staff.

Reactions

❖ Transient blanching due to capillary vasoconstriction.

Ametop cream

❖ Mixture of Lignocaine and Prilocaine.

❖ Action: acts by topical vasodilation.

Application

❖ Not to be used on infants under one month and preterm babies.

❖ Apply cream for a minimum of 30 minutes prior to venepuncture, 45 minutes to venous cannulation.

❖ Avoid contact with eyes, mouth and mucosal surfaces.

Removal

❖ Remove gauze swab, site can be accessed up to four to six hours following removal of excess cream.

❖ Observe skin condition following procedure and note any reactions and record in the nursing notes and inform medical staff.

Reactions

❖ Localised erythema, oedema, itching due to vasodilatation action of amethocaine.

Adaptation for home care

● Apply as in hospital.

Best practice

❖ It is advisable to remove cream before the child is taken to theatre to reduce the possibility of localised reaction and to help keep the child calm in the anaesthetic room.

Research and relevant articles

Lawson RA, Smart NG *et al* (1995) Evaluation of amethocaine gel preparation for percutaneous analgesia before venous cannulation in children. *British Journal of Anaesthesia* **75**(3): 282–5

Woolfson AD, McCafferty DF, Boston V (1990) Clinical experience with novel percutaneous amethocane preparation: prevention of pain due to venepuncture in children. *British Journal of Clinical Pharmacology* **30**: 273–9

Lee JJ, Rubin A (1993) Emla cream and its current uses. *British Journal of Hospital Medicine* **50**(8): 463–6

Watson K *Emla Cream.* For further information contact the head of medical information at Astra Pharmaceuticals Ltd

See *Appendix III*

Nursing notes

Trolley cleansing

Definition: The cleansing of a trolley used in a clinical procedure

Purpose: To ensure a clean or sterile working surface as required.

Equipment required

- Trolley
- Liquid detergent
- Hot water
- Paper towels
- 70% isopropyl alcohol wipes (as required).

Nursing interventions

- Wash whole trolley from top to bottom with hot water and liquid detergent once a day
- Remove excess detergent (with clear water) and continue until all detergent is removed
- Dry trolley surfaces using paper towels
- Prior to each individual procedure wipe trolley surface with 70% isopropyl alcohol wipe and allow to dry, completely.

Adaptation for home care

- The principles of the above procedures can be applied in the home setting. Plastic trays rather than trolleys may be more convenient.

See *Appendix III*

> *Nursing notes*

Clinical governance and nursing audit

The concept of audit has become embedded in the culture of the NHS over the last decade as a means of evaluating performance through the systematic analysis of clinical practice, including the procedures for delivering care, the use of resources, and the resulting outcomes in terms of effectiveness and quality of life for the patient (DoH, 1989; Malby, 1995). More specifically nursing audit can be defined as:

> *... part of the audit cycle of quality assurance. It incorporates the systematic and critical analysis by nurses, midwives and health visitors, in conjunction with other staff, of the planning, delivery and evaluation of nursing and midwifery care, in terms of their use of resources and the outcomes for patients/clients, and introduces appropriate change in response to that analysis.*

(NHS ME, 1991)

Audit therefore is a cycle of activity which systematically reviews practice against agreed criteria. The process includes identification of specific problems and potential solutions. An associated action plan is produced to facilitate the required changes in practice prior to a further review. A key to this process is the agreement of the criteria considered to represent 'good' practice. Ideally these criteria which lead on to the development of universal standards will be research based (Malby, 1995). In instances where evidence is limited a combination of available evidence and expert opinion should be used.

With the publication of the White Paper *The New NHS: Modern, Dependable* (DoH, 1997) the principles of efficiency and excellence are key features for the organization of the service and refer to the delivery of best evidence-based practice, developed in the most cost effective manner. This new emphasis on quality of care through the development of standards and guidelines is laid out in *A First Class Service: Quality in the New NHS* (DoH, 1998) and places renewed emphasis on the importance of auditing current practice and planning for change through a system of clinical governance. There will be national guidance through the work of two new systems. The National Service Framework which will issue recommendations for patterns of service and the National Institute for Clinical Excellence which will be responsible for providing guidance on clinical and cost effectiveness (Crinson, 1999).

The main aim of clinical governance is a marriage of national standards and clinical judgement to promote a consistent approach to the quality and cost effectiveness of locally delivered care, underpinned by the concepts of lifelong learning and continuing professional development (DoH, 1998).

There are five main components to the concept of clinical governance (NHSE North Thames Regional Office, 1998). These are:

- **Clinical audit** – rather than the previous uni-professional approach to audit a multi-professional model to reflect the combined contribution of a number of professionals to patient care is advocated. Key to the success of such an approach will be a culture and environment which promotes open discussion and review followed by agreed changes in existing practice (Malby, 1995).
- **Clinical effectiveness** – here the emphasis is on the use of evidence-based care. This requires all healthcare professionals to develop the skills of critical appraisal to enable the interpretation and assessment of the available evidence in terms of the individual patients needs and any agreed standards of care (Crinson, 1999).

- **Clinical risk management** – aiming at reducing the likelihood of adverse events through the identification of potential risk. By using a systematic process to assess and review the 'probability' of an adverse situation decisions can be made to prevent or minimise the risk and to develop contingency plans.
- **Quality assurance** – through clinical audit and data collection from a variety of sources to reflect the different dimensions of healthcare and delivery, standards can be set and monitored on a regular basis to assess the organisations progress or maintenance of these standards.
- **Continuing professional development, education and training** – to support the changing face of the NHS and service delivery, continuing education, training and development is crucial to the delivery of safe and effective care and therefore the achievement of the goals of clinical governance.

Individual Trusts are responsible for ensuring through their system of clinical governance that standards which reflect the national guidance are set and maintained while individual healthcare professionals will be accountable and responsible for the quality of care that they deliver (DoH,1998). It is for this reason that the guidelines in this manual have been developed.

Guidelines represent one stage in the total quality cycle by setting the local standard against which existing practice can be measured. These guidelines, focusing on aspects of clinical care, must be seen as a dynamic entity in that they must be reviewed and up-dated on a regular basis to reflect changes in thinking and practice supported by up-to-date literature and research findings. At the present time much nursing practice has developed incrementally with little scientific basis, therefore these guidelines are based on a review of existing literature and expert/specialist nursing opinion. As clearer national guidance becomes available these guidelines will be up-dated to reflect this. In support of this evidence-based agenda there is a central recognition of the need to develop a strategy for nursing research and development which will include the development of nurses' critical appraisal skills and research expertise and the active support of funded research into nursing practice (DoH, 1999).

The value of developing guidelines for nursing practice lies in the consistency of approach to patient care from a qualitative and educative perspective. Guidelines such as those contained within this manual provide an excellent platform for the teaching of clinical skills, encompassing an holistic approach to care rather than one that is purely skills based. While it is important that nurses have competent skills, the context in which the skill is performed is of equal importance to the quality of patient care delivered. A nurse who is practically skilled but lacks the knowledge and understanding to use the skill appropriately, or to safely adapt the accepted procedure to meet the individual needs of the patient, is as incompetent as the nurse who has the knowledge but is unable to carry out the necessary task in the accepted manner.

To ensure that current practice reflects the recommendations laid out in the relevant guideline a periodic observational audit should take place whereby the care/practice delivered by a nurse is measured against the guideline. This observation may be undertaken either as a self-audit or peer-audit process, however to ensure a consistent approach it is recommended that a standard tool is used. The tool included in this chapter represents an approach for use at the Birmingham Children's Hospital NHS Trust. It aims to encapsulate the philosophy of child and family centered care established within the Trust.

It is recommended that a peer audit approach is used as this provides opportunity for feedback on performance, linking the practice to the overall care of the patient and stimulating intellectual discussion of the approach used. This discussion is an essential component of the development of nursing only if key issues are fed back to the originators of the guideline to contribute to the review process. Comments and suggestions which remain only between the observers are quickly lost, contributing nothing to the body of nursing knowledge and advancement of care.

Following the audit and resulting discussion areas, if there is a need to improve or change practice then either amendments to the individual nurses practice or the guideline can be made before undertaking a further audit as part of the process of continuous improvement.

The educational value of undertaking an audit of practice cannot be underestimated. Firstly, the feedback process should be viewed and conducted in a positive way to enable both parties to learn from the interaction between practitioner and observer. This process encourages the development of an even greater understanding of the rationale which underpins the guideline. From a student nurse's perspective this process should facilitate a greater degree of confidence in their ability to deliver sound nursing care. The audit process also provides an opportunity to feed back results to educational institutions regarding the relevance and effectiveness of curriculum content, thus promoting discussion for future course development. It also provides an opportunity for the organisation to assure itself of the competence of its employees and to identify future training needs.

The generic audit tool which is illustrated in *Figure 3.1* is one example that can be used by individuals or peers to consistently assess the standard of nursing care delivered.

References

Castledine G (1999) Professional misconduct case studies. *British Journal of Nursing* **8**(7): 419

Crinson I (1999) Clinical governance: the new NHS, new responsibilities? *British Journal of Nursing* **8**(7): 449–53

Department of Health (1997) *The New NHS: Modern, Dependable.* HMSO, London

Department of Health (1998) *A First Class Service: Quality in the New NHS Health Services.* HMSO, London

Department of Health (1989) *Working for Patients.* HMSO, London

Department of Health (1999) *Making a Difference.* HMSO, London

NHS ME (1991) *A Framework of Audit for Nursing Services.* HMSO, London

NHSE North Thames Regional Office (1998a) *Clinical Governance in North Thames: A Paper for Discussion and Consultation.* June 1998, *Department of Public Health, London*

Malby B (1995) *Clinical Audit for Nurses and Therapists.* Scutari Press, London

Figure 3.1: Generic Audit Tool Clinical Nursing Guidelines

1.   Title of procedure

2.   Ward/Dept: 3.   Grade of nurse:

4.   Age of patient: 5.   How long did the procedure take:

6.   **Was the manual referred to:**

Prior to the procedure   ☐   Comments:

During the procedure   ☐

After the procedure   ☐

Not at all   ☐

7.   Who explained the procedure to the

Child/adolescent   **Parent/carer**

Nurse carrying out the procedure   ☐   Nurse carrying out the procedure   ☐

Other   ☐   Other   ☐

N/A Please state reason: N/A Please state reason:

Please specify:

8.   Was the child's/parent's understanding of the procedure assessed

Child/adolescent   **Parent/carer**

Yes   ☐   Yes   ☐

No   ☐   No   ☐

N/A Please state reason: N/A Please state reason:

Comments:

9.   How did the nurse assess the understanding of

Child/adolescent

Parent/carer

10. Were any available teaching tools used to explain the procedure

Yes   ☐

No   ☐

If N/A Please state reason:

Please specify:

11. Did the child/adolescent and the parent/carer agree for the procedure to begin

Child/adolescent   **Parent/carer**

Yes   ☐   Yes   ☐

No   ☐   No   ☐

N/A   ☐   N/A   ☐

If N/A Please state reason:

Comments:

12. Did the nurse prepare the procedure following the manual guidelines

Yes, all of the guidelines were followed   ☐

Most of the guidelines were followed, but some were N/A   ☐

No, all of the guidelines were not followed   ☐

Comments:

13. Did the nurse incorporate the procedure into the child/adolescent's care plan

Yes   ☐

No   ☐

N/A   ☐

If N/A Please state reason:

Comments:

14. Was the parent/carer able to stay during the procedure

Yes   ☐

No   ☐

If not specify:

15. If baseline observations were necessary prior to the procedure were they recorded

Yes, all of the baseline observations were recorded   ☐

Some of them were recorded, but some were omitted   ☐

No, none were recorded   ☐

Observations not necessary   ☐

Comments:

16.   If it was necessary to monitor observations during the procedure were they recorded

Yes, all were recorded ☐

Some were recorded, but some were omitted ☐

No, none were recorded ☐

Not necessary ☐

Comments:

17.   If it was necessary to monitor observations following the procedure were they recorded

Yes, all were recorded ☐

Some were recorded, but some were omitted ☐

No, none were recorded ☐

Not necessary ☐.

Comments:

18.   During the procedure did the child/adolescent or parent/carer become distressed

Child/adolescent		**Parent/carer**	
Yes	☐	Yes	☐
No	☐	No	☐

Briefly explain:

19a   If the procedure was interrupted at any point was this due to

Parental stress ☐

Child/adolescent stress ☐

Complications ☐

Other, please state ☐

Comments:

19b.   Was the medical team informed

Yes ☐

No ☐

N/A ☐

Comments:

Appendix I: Effectiveness of pH measurements in predicting feeding tubes placement

To increase probability of obtaining accurate results with pH paper, the following points should be kept in mind for pH testing:

- Immediately before aspirating fluid for pH testing, put air down to clear the tube of other substances
- Remember some enteral feeds in use are acidic in nature
- Remember some children not receiving acid-inhibiting agents (H2 — receptor antagonists or Omperazole); pH values of aspirate from gastric site will range from 0–4; intestinal site ranges will be greater than 4. Blue litmus paper will be effective in these situations
- Children receiving acid-inhibiting agents (defined H2 — receptor antagonist or Omperzole) will require yellow litmus paper to be used
- Nurses are responsible for verifying correct feeding tube position. Failure to detect respiratory placement before initiating tube feeding can produce lethal pulmonary complications
- Any difficult or unsuccessful nasogastric intubation or bloody aspirate from the tube, complaints of chest or upper abdominal pain should heighten the awareness of tube misplacement
- **Important** — if tube placement is suspected to have caused trauma, a chest x-ray should be done immediately, preferably with the tube still in place if this does not impair the child's breathing. Leaving the tube in place is important because it may have entered the pleural space and its removal would result in pneumothorax
- **High risk patient** — nasogastric tubes can be displayed easily in children who have difficulty in swallowing or have an endotracheal tube in place
  - X-ray confirmation of tube placement may be necessary. NB. both aspiration and x-ray confirmation techniques only confirm the position at the instant they are taken
  - As tubes can easily and repeatedly relocate, it is essential that aspiration to confirm placement is used when starting feeding and repeated four-hourly if continuous feeds are in use.

Important additional information to check placement

Correct measuring of the length of the nasogastric tube to be inserted is essential to ensure correct placement. Strobels formula determines the oesophageal junction sphincter. This could potentially be adapted as a second check to confirm the nursing estimated interpretation of the length of tube to be inserted by adding 3–4cms on to the formula to determine gastric antrium.

Strobels formula to calculate aesophageal

Oesophageal sphincter can be accurately predicted be employing the following respective equations:

EL Oesophageal length (cms) = 6.7 + 0.226 (H+) cm.

To determine gastric antrium 3–4cms to be added to above formula

Reference

Strobel CT, Byrne WJ, Ament ME, Euler AR (1979) Correlation of oesophageal lengths in children with height: Application to the Turtle test without prior oesophageal. *Journal of Paediatrics* **94**(1): 81–4

Appendix II: Guide to categories of isolation and source isolation categories

Categories of isolation	Single room required	Gloves required	Apron required
Respiratory	Yes Door must be closed NB. Patients with the same infection may be cohorted	For all activities that involve a risk of exposure to respiratory secretions, or handling potentially contaminated equipment	WHITE or BLUE plastic aprons for all activities that involved a risk of exposure to respiratory secretions or handling contaminated equipment
Excretion/secretion/ blood isolation	Not always required The Infection Control Team will advise on individual cases	For all activities that involve patient contact, or handling of potentially contaminated equipment	WHITE or BLUE plastic aprons for all activities that involve a risk of exposure to faeces, or handling contaminated equipment
Enteric isolation	Preferred, but less important for infants confined to their own cot	For all activities that involve patient contact, or handling of potentially contaminated equipment	WHITE or BLUE plastic aprons for all activities that involve a risk of exposure to faeces, or handling contaminated equipment
Skin/wound isolation	Usually required Door must be kept closed	Whenever entering the room	Must be worn whenever entering the room. WHITE or BLUE aprons should be used for alla activities except serving food, when a YELLOW apron should be worn.

Source isolation categories			
Disease	**Isolation precautions**	**Disease**	**Isolation precautions**
AIDS	Excretion/secretion/blood	Measles	Respiratory
Anthrax	STRICT	Meningococcal disease	Respiratory
Chicken pox	Respiratory excretion/secretion (vesicle fluid)	Mumps	Respiratory
Cholera	Enteric	Pediculosis	Skin/wound
Cytomegalovirus	Excretion/secretion (urine, respiratory secretions)	Pertussis	Respiratory
Diptheria	STRICT	Plague	STRICT
Gastro-enteritis, bacterial or protozoal	Enteric	Poliomyelitis, acute	Respiratory enteric
Gastro-enteritis, viral	Enteric respiratory	Psittacosis	Respiratory
Gonococcal opthalmia	Excretion/secretion (eye discharge)	Rabies	STRICT
Group A streptococcus (Streptococcus pyogenes)	Skin/wound respiratory	Rubella (congenital)	Respiratory
Haemophilus influenzae Type B (Hib) disease	Respiratory	Scabies	Excretion/secretion (urine)
Hand, foot and mouth	Respiratory excretion/secretion (vesicle fluid)	Shingles	Skin/wound
Hepatitis A	Enteric	Tuberculosis	Excretion/secretion (vesicle fluid)
Hepatitis B	Excretion/secretion/blood	Typhoid/paratyphoid fever	Respiratory
Hepatitis C	Excretion/secretion/blood	Viral haemorrhagic fever	Enteric excretion/secretion (urine)
Hepatitis D	Excretion/secretion/blood	Yellow fever	STRICT
Hepatitis E	Enteric	Infections with multi-resistant bacteria, eg. MRSA	STRICT
Herpes simplex virus	Excretion/secretion (vesicle fluid)		Seek advice from ICT
Leptospirosis	Excretion/secretion (urine)		
Leprosy	Excretion/secretion (nasal discharge)		

Appendix III

The following form is attached to the individual protocols supplied by the Birmingham Children's Hospital NHS Trust.

Originated by:	
Approved by:	
Date of development:	Review date:
Circulation to:	

SOUTH-EAST ASIAN CURRIES

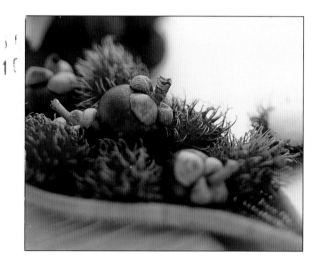

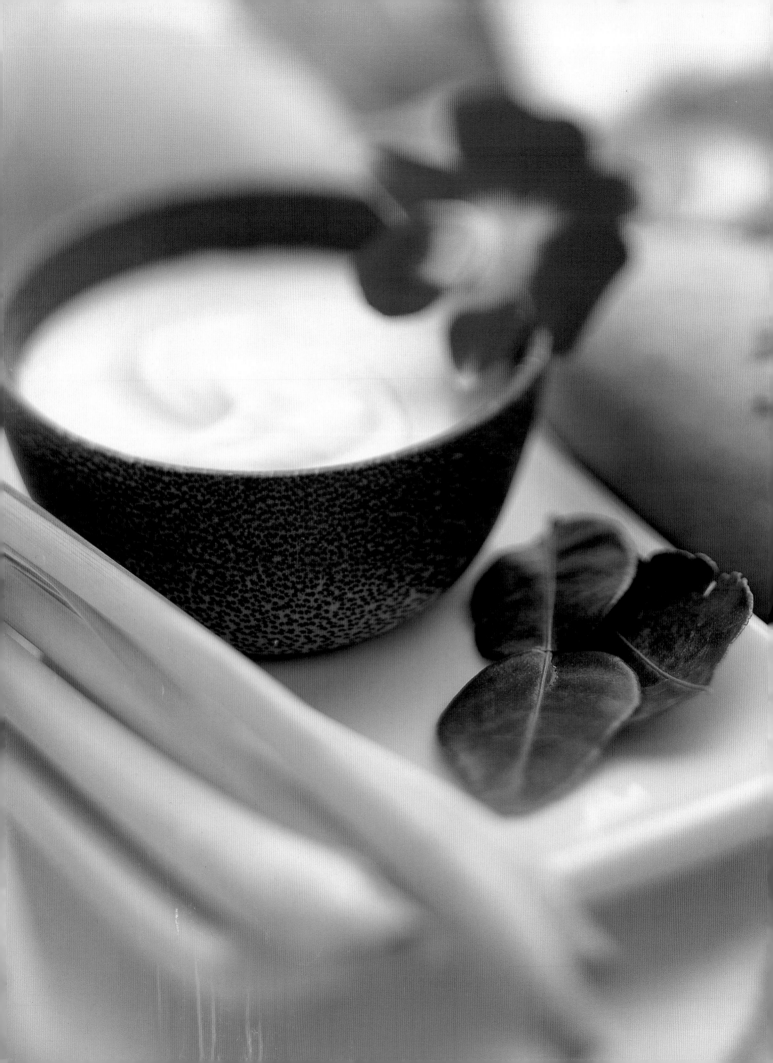